On a Lark!

Creative Movement for Children

Featuring the Essential **ABC** Building Blocks of Movement:
Alignment, **B**reathing and **C**entering

Written by Larkin Barnett, B.A., M.A., Dance

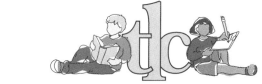

Teaching & Learning Company

1204 Buchanan St., P.O. Box 10
Carthage, IL 62321-0010

This book belongs to

_____

Copyright © 2008, Larkin Barnett

Published by the Teaching & Learning Company

ISBN No. 10: 1-57310-547-3

ISBN No. 13: 978-1-57310-547-7

Printing No. 987654321

Teaching & Learning Company
1204 Buchanan St., P.O. Box 10
Carthage, IL 62321-0010

Table of Contents

A Is for Alignment

B Is for Breathing

C Is for Centering

Introduction

by Dr. Dot Richardson, Vice Chair, President's Council on Physical Fitness and Sports and Two-Time Olympic Gold Medalist

As a two-time Olympic gold medalist, orthopedic surgeon and current Vice Chair of the President's Council on Physical Fitness and Sports, I sincerely hope that classroom teachers, movement educators, parents and therapists will take advantage of this resource to help children learn how to use their bodies in functional and expressive movement.

Larkin Barnett is an expert on functional training having written *Functional Fitness* for adults. Now generations of children will benefit from the secrets to a healthy life-style through her latest work. As you know, functional movement relates to work, play, fitness and sports. Larkin's program introduces children to the building blocks inherent in any movement arena.

You know, few people ever discover the key to health—a positive mind-set. Athletes often use positive visualization skills to improve the mechanics of their event. As a young girl, I visualized myself on the podium winning an Olympic gold medal for my country. Twenty-seven years later I found myself living that vision, that dream. I can only imagine the impact Ms. Barnett's visual imagery will have on encouraging children's natural use of their imagination to dream big and live their Olympic life.

The emphasis of Larkin's program focuses primarily on expressive movement, which involves mastery over the body in all its varieties. Body awareness builds a child's confidence. This self-esteem prepares them for participation in sports and helps them create healthy active habits for a lifetime. Children move at their own pace. Instead of doing a fitness task or winning a race, they learn to structure their own dances. They learn to communicate their own feelings about the world through problem-solving in combination with creative self-expression. The child is doing, acting, being—and having fun!

In today's world, it is becoming more and more significant to merely push the chairs back in a classroom and let children move, especially with fewer physical education classes and the rise in childhood obesity. This simple, comprehensive guide makes the joy and satisfaction of movement exploration a vital part of a well-balanced physical education program. There are many opportunities in the form of academic-oriented movement lessons to enhance the total educative process. The combination of building a movement vocabulary is tied into academic enrichment. The children are introduced to the power of the mind/body connection. After all, children explore their world first through their rich imagination and five senses. These are versatile, simple and fun activity options for the classroom, gymnasium, fitness, dance, home and therapeutic environments.

It is apparent to everyone that many of our children lack the joy found in total body rhythmic action, having been restrained by push buttons and computers. They are content to be spectators, to sit on the sidelines, to watch the game on TV. When motor activities play no part in life, a child does not develop socially and becomes sluggish nutritionally. For a child, it is a delight to skip with joyous abandonment. Expressive movement is a rich resource for energy release and communication—and it is a biological necessity. Mastery over the body's movement relates to physical as well as emotional and mental development.

Through Larkin's Creative Movement program, children make it a priority to chart their progress. Children become motivated and inspired. They build discipline through consistency, which is the most important ingredient to attaining goals. Enjoy the adventure and excitement that this program will bring to many. Keep making a difference in the lives of others.

Best regards,

Dot Richardson, M.D.
Vice Chair, President's Council on Physical Fitness and Sports
Director and Medical Director
National Training Center
Olympic Gold Medalist—Softball (1996 and 2000)

I'd like to extend an invitation to everyone to join and help children join the free program offered by the President's Council on Physical Fitness and Sports called the President's Challenge (www.presidentschallenge.org). I'd like to see the joy in the children's faces when they participate in Larkin's program, as well as receive the President's Award!

Foreword

by Dr. Quentin L. Van Meter, M.D., Pediatric Endocrinology Specialist

What an inspiration it was to open the cover of *On a Lark!* to find such a refreshing and exhilarating avenue for children to follow on their way to a life-style of fitness and emotional growth. Obesity has become everyone's favorite epidemic, with the laying of blame on bad environmental influences. In this book on Creative Movement for Children, Larkin Barnett provides a road map for children of all sizes and shapes to move away from sedentary, constricting habits that promote obesity. What a wonderful world it would be if all children moved themselves through space with confidence, uninhibited by fear of being judged for not having moved in "the right way." Without falling prey to the school of thought that promotes mediocrity for the sake of making students feel better about themselves, Ms. Barnett promotes a constantly open-ended routine that stokes the spirit of her students and makes them blossom any way they can. Imagine having a generation of spirited, unabashedly creative kids taking the natural steps beyond Creative Movement to become impassioned pre-teens who feel compelled to move their bodies effectively in all endeavors. Confidence ensues that helps these kids see the bridge between physical exertion and sound nutrition, and the beat goes on.

The basic ABCs of Alignment, Breathing and Centering, which are pulled from the Pilates philosophy, are the proven core of the "curriculum" that Ms. Barnett outlines so well. Adapted from her established treatise for adults, *Functional Fitness*, these principles, which were the obvious building blocks of her adult program, and which are responsible for its success, are woven into her program for children. They are discussed but do not detract from the lightheart-edness and whimsical attractiveness of her child-centered program. They are an invisible foundation, and as one who has decided to try out the *Functional Fitness* program, I can vouch for these ABCs as sound concepts.

The layout of this workbook takes away any second thoughts a teacher might have about not having enough time to make the lesson plan work. The end of each chapter is designed to clarify the progress of each lesson. I could not help but imagine how fun it would be to be a "fly on the wall" while watching the teacher and pupils create these masterpieces of movement literally anywhere there is an open space. Within the time constraints of a small recess period or a wide open afternoon of an otherwise bland after-school program, *On a Lark!* makes hay with the creative spirit of children who would otherwise sit quietly and marginalize themselves for fear of taking a chance and coming up short of someone's expectations. Children who experience the joy of learning to control their own bodies then take on the bigger challenge of moving with purpose in work and play, and the next thing you know, they grow more and more comfortable in their skin as people dedicated to personalized physical fitness for the rest of their lives. This gives hope to those of us who see children as the greatest resource we have on this planet of ours. Let's get moving!

Dr. Quentin L. Van Meter, M.D.
Pediatric Endocrinology Specialist

Preface

The *ABCs* of Movement for Children

Children are naturally at home in their bodies. From the first step to running and jumping on the playground, children love being in motion. *On a Lark! Creative Movement for Children* channels the energy and creativity of children into the essential "ABC" building blocks of Pilates training.

This new approach to the ABCs of Alignment, Breathing and Centering does not require any formal dance or Pilates training. The book's simple, well-organized lesson plans make the principles of movement come alive for children. Specific lessons enhance and support academic learning. Children can even learn the alphabet while using the ABCs of Pilates movement. Creative Movement is an essential educational experience for all ages. Preschool, kindergarten, elementary and secondary school children learn a specific movement language. For boys and girls ages 4-10, this simple approach deals with the movement potential of the body in varied, daring and challenging ways, thereby making dance a sought-after activity for all children. Learning takes place through practical problem-solving. Children are given easy, fun opportunities to experiment with movement ideas. The movement progression is sequential, culminating in the final dance in each lesson, which has a beginning, middle and end.

Younger children perceive, organize and understand the world primarily through their physical senses. In dance, they learn how to "speak" through their bodies and therefore become aware of body language and its relationship to words. In Creative Movement, children express themselves by clearly communicating their unique feelings about the specific assignment, as well as interpreting their view of the world.

On a Lark! began through the author's interaction with a curious four-year-old boy named Brandon.

During the course of baby-sitting for Brandon, I would perform dance stretches, which Brandon began to copy. Soon, Brandon and I were off on a joint journey of discovery, exploring the fitness training principles of Joseph Pilates and the dance movement vocabulary of Rudolf Laban. Brandon enthusiastically participated even as he added his own take on the subject.

Brandon's parents remarked on noticeable changes as he became more expressive. They quickly discovered he not only had an extensive repertoire of moves but also that he was more verbal, with an expanded vocabulary.

On a Lark! begins with an exploration of the elements of dance. Once grasped, the child combines the elements utilizing space, force and time. Creative Movement involves a clearly defined body of knowledge, which can be learned, explored, and structured.

Creative Movement for Children is a special kind of dance instruction. Most dance instruction is burdensome to children. They are often asked to express a specific image, such as a flower or even a piece of music. Or they are asked to perform structured movements requiring tremendous discipline.

However, in Creative Dance, a movement educator uses the language of Laban exclusively. This allows children the opportunity to explore, experiment and invent. Children learn the names of movements and how to make simple combinations. Factors of time, space and force are added for diversity to increase kinesthetic awareness. The result is an exhilarating sensation of control and confidence. Children achieve proper biological development while their hunger for movement is satisfied.

Creative Movement allows children to:

- Explore, experiment and invent.

- Learn names of movements and simple combinations.

- Increase their kinesthetic awareness by realizing factors of time, space and force.

- Discover a great deal about their bodies, language, thoughts and imagination.

- Develop a "can do" attitude.

Because dance engages the mind, body and spirit, it allows children to discover a great deal about their body, language, thoughts and imagination. They not only learn tangible skills and develop a "can do" attitude, but they also learn intangibles, like an intuitive sense of body language. These are all confidence-builders, which will serve children well as they mature.

Dance is unlike any other art medium. The dancer and his or her creation are one. Unlike singing or drawing, dancing involves the total child. Dance is the most intimate expressive medium. It develops self-confidence and identity.

This book is written for all children in schools and day-care centers, as well as those who are home-schooled. The simplicity of the program fits into classroom breaks, academic curriculum, elementary physical education programs, recess, therapeutic settings and structured child care activities. By incorporating movement experiences into educational activities, interaction with children is deepened, thereby stimulating both the right and left sides of the brain. The succinct text, guide boxes and new approach to the Pilates principles and Laban elements of movement will help those who work with children to incorporate Creative Movement into other learning and enrichment activities. Key words are contained in the Visual Aid Guide Boxes. Write them on the chalkboard; the children will then connect the word with the action, and they are off on a lark!

How to Use This Book

Children initially relate to the world around them and communicate to others through their bodies. This program is an easy, fun way to help children continue to make important connections between their bodies and learning. This program is more scientific than merely being told to move in any way you wish. There are lessons that correspond to classroom subjects such as science, arithmetic, vocabulary, anatomy, geometry and storytelling.

Visual Aid Guide Boxes

You will find the Visual Aid Guide Boxes at the back of the book. These boxes contain a user-friendly summary of the lesson plans. To simplify your preparation for each lesson, post the words from this box on the chalkboard. This will cut your preparation time in half. Children can also increase their vocabulary by seeing the words.

Be dramatic as you call out these action words for the children to follow.

These boxes will also help you to "get a feel" for a particular Creative Movement session.

The *On a Lark!* Recipe for Teaching Creative Movement for Children

This is a user-friendly teaching guide. *Creative Movement for Children* is a dynamic blend of the essential movement concepts from Joseph Pilates and Rudolf Laban. These movement principles and elements are also the same essential ingredients found in dance, athletics, yoga and the martial arts.

This "recipe" combines the main movement concepts and action words from these various disciplines.

They provide the *purpose* for movement. Children quickly learn the vocabulary to accompany the movements. In the beginning, specific movements are directed by the teacher. Then children are called upon to move increasingly on their own. They make decisions and solve problems. Specific words become points of departure for movement explorations. These action words also help children access the artistry, inspiration and joy of moving.

The *On a Lark!* "Recipes"

Joseph Pilates Principles of Movement

Ingredients

The ABCs ➔ **Alignment • Breathing • Centering**

Method
Mix the principles of movement to clarify the fundamentals of how the body functions. They are like a well-stocked pantry. These are the keys to success in Pilates, fitness, dance, sports, martial arts, yoga and stress management.

Rudolf Laban's Elements of Movement

Ingredients

Time	Attitude	Fast	⟷	Slow
Space	Quality	Directions	▬▬	Levels
		Pathways	▬▬	Range
Force	Effort	Heavy	⟷	Light
	Weight	Strong	⟷	Soft
Shape	Design	Round	⟷	Pointed
		Large	⟷	Small
Flow	Energy	Free	⟷	Bound

Method

Stir in the delicious elements that bring out the qualities of movement. They extend children's movement possibilities. For example, children explore spatial options—diagonal pathways, twists, turns, spirals, including the areas behind the body—like the motion of a pitcher throwing a baseball. The emphasis is on total body spatial exploration, three-dimensional mobility and expression.

The Moving Body and Its Relationship to Kinetic Energy

Ingredients

Gravity	⟷	The Body	⟷	Energy
Muscular Contraction			⟷	Release
Balance			⟷	Weight Shifts
Rhythm				
Controlled Momentum				

Method

Add the remaining *spicy* **kinetics** to bring out the exciting artistry of movement. These are essential ingredients in sports and dance. For example, the weight shifts in basketball and the timing of a serve in tennis. They create a greater potential for feeling the joy of moving.

Serving Suggestion

A basic movement education is excellent for the physiological, mental, emotional and social development of children from ages 4 to 10.

Recommendations

Parents, teachers, day-care workers and therapists: Familiarize yourselves with this Recipe because it contains the materials for dance exploration. *Follow these guide boxes located at the beginning of each lesson.

Kinetics

At the foundation of modern dance expression is the constant awareness between the body's internal state of muscular tension and the external force of gravity. Children will automatically be introduced to the kinesthetic "feel" or sensory experience of movement in Creative Movement. For example, they demonstrate contrasting relationships to **gravity**. The teacher asks them to move while feeling like heavy clay or a light feather. They are asked to **contract all of their muscles**, to "freeze in a shape." Children explore their bodies' **weight shifts and balance** while stepping over an imaginary rain puddle. While **changing rhythms and speed** they run, collapse, spin and jump up. Children dash through space tracing gigantic curvy pathways while feeling the physical sensation of **controlled momentum**.

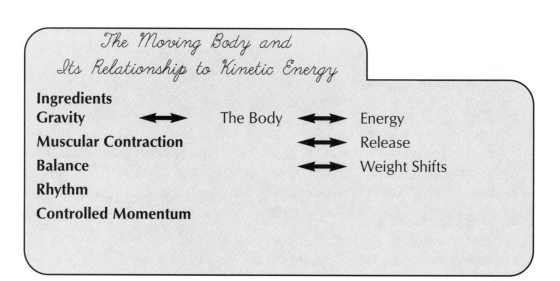

Kinetics

noun:
Scientific study of forces and energy on the moving body.

adjective:
Example: "Modern dance has been called kinetic pantomime."

The Moving Body and Its Relationship to Kinetic Energy

Ingredients
Gravity ⟷ The Body ⟷ Energy
Muscular Contraction ⟷ Release
Balance ⟷ Weight Shifts
Rhythm
Controlled Momentum

Movement Vocabulary Is the Key to Success

The principles, elements and kinetic aspects of movement are a body of knowledge that can be taught to either a child or adult. Modern dancers have utilized this vocabulary for years to analyze movement and create dances. When you use this terminology exclusively, you are providing a purpose for movement exploration.

Three Main Movement Categories in Creative Movement

Body Parts	Locomotor Movements That Carry the Body from One Place to Another	Non-Locomotor Movements Performed in One Place Within the Space
head	walk	bend
neck	run	stretch
arms	skip	twist
shoulders	gallop	swing
elbows	jump	push
wrists	hop	pull
hands	leap	shake
fingers	slide	collapse
back		rise
trunk		
hips		
legs		
knees		
ankles		
feet		
toes		

It is the endless combinations of these movements and the application of the elements of time, space, force, shape and flow that make up the materials for movement experimentation and the invention of dances.

For example, the following demonstrates how to combine running with each category of the elements of movement:

"Run as fast as you can throughout the space. Run while changing directions. Try running forward, backwards and sideways. Run on your tiptoes and on a low level. Trace curvy and straight pathways while running. Explore a run that feels either heavy, light, strong or soft. Make round, pointed, large and small shapes with your body while running. Add loose upper-body swings to your runs. Run like heavy clay."

The Elements of Movement and Their Contrasts

Ingredients

Time	Attitude	Fast	⟷	Slow
Space	Quality	Directions:		Forward/Backwards, Sideways, Up/Down,
		Levels:		High/Medium/Low
		Pathways:		Straight/Curvy, Zigzags/Turning
		Range:		Big/Little
Force	Effort	Heavy	⟷	Light
	Weight	Strong	⟷	Soft
Shape	Design	Round	⟷	Pointed
		Large	⟷	Small
		Wide	⟷	Narrow
Flow	Energy	Free Flow/	⟷	Bound Control/
		Loose	⟷	Tight

The Teacher's Role in Guiding Movement Experiences

Your first task is to identify the main elements to explore during a particular lesson. Structure the lesson through **direction, suggestion, questions** and **challenges.**

The following are examples:

> **Direction:** Skip from one end of the room to the other.
>
> **Suggestion:** Try to skip while turning.
>
> **Question:** Can you skip fast and then gradually make it very slow?
>
> **Challenge:** Find a way to skip forward and then backward.

This discipline and structure promote creativity. They enable children to discover a variety of solutions to the tasks presented.

- **Provide ample time to refine and practice the chosen solution.** In time, children will perform movements with more control, innovation and complexity. They will discover through improvisation how to choreograph mini-dances. It is important in Creative Movement to eventually offer plenty of opportunities for children to make their own decisions. They will discover there are several ways to perform every movement.

- **At first, you will use more words.** As the lessons progress, children will require less instruction.

- **Challenge them with a lot of variety.**

- **Experiment with a supportive, firm, natural and dramatic voice.** The quality of your voice builds, develops and draws each movement exploration to a close. Your voice is your most potent teaching aid.

- **Be aware of your posture and energize your own body.** The teacher does not dance with children. Sometimes you will need to physically clarify an activity. Move freely about the room in order to really see all children.

- **Teachers who work with higher grade levels may wish to omit certain activities; challenge students by increasing the level of difficulty.** Even upper-grade children whose movement backgrounds are limited enjoy repeating the skills and exploring combinations.

Teacher's Tip

In order to cut your preparation time in half, each lesson is also summarized for you in the Visual Aid Guide Boxes at the end of the book.

Lesson Structure

A series of planned lessons may be impractical. You may have to decide how to fit them into classroom or recess activities. It is also beneficial to use movement words during child care activities. View these lessons as movement ideas that you have at your fingertips. They can be flexible. You and your students can plan and explore together. Your hands-on experience will provide your best guideline. You may find that you will develop your own lessons to meet the specific needs and interests of the children.

Lesson plans have been structured to help children understand movement elements and principles. These lessons create a cohesive educational dance experience.

The second lesson in Chapter 2 begins by calling out the children's names, accompanied by rhythmic clapping.

Introduce them to an understanding of their own "self-space." Children progress to learn the essential movement concept of stillness. They practice finding various body shapes and then freezing them.

This is followed by an exploration of isolated body parts, the entire body and locomotor movements such as running, jumping, skipping, hopping and galloping. Finally, children combine a variety of these elements of movement.

Example of Lesson Structure

1. Call out children's names, accompanied by rhythmic clapping.
2. Introduce children to their own "self-space."
3. Introduce the concept of stillness. Practice finding various body shapes and then freezing them.
4. Isolate body parts, the entire body and locomotor movements. Then combine a variety of these elements of movement.
5. Each child creates a "Good-Bye Dance" at the end of every lesson.

Each child creates his or her own "Good-Bye Dance" at the end of every lesson. They learn to structure the improvised elements of movement explored during that lesson. Children are encouraged to problem-solve. They think of the movement elements in terms of sequential form. **The dance has a beginning, middle and end.** This enhances a child's ability to structure any form of communication. The creation of a final dance is similar to learning to form a sentence, paragraph, story, musical score or piece of choreography. The "Good-Bye Dance" includes a definite starting shape. This proceeds with action and arrives at a point of completion in a frozen shape. Children's physical, mental and emotional skills help them fulfill this goal. This exercise improves efficiency in attacking new problems. The result is an ever-broadening cycle of learning. The final dance is also the child's opportunity to demonstrate his or her individuality in response to the specific lesson. It is a moment to perform and shine.

Creating his own dance teaches a child how to organize his thinking, communicate, create and problem-solve. It may also be the child's first introduction to dance as a performance art. It is both audience-oriented and movement-oriented. You will divide the class in half. Each group is given a turn to either watch or perform. Children feel more comfortable inventing and showing their final dances in a group. Due to time constraints, the class can also perform together.

The structure of a lesson is simple. Begin by introducing the movement words and concepts for a particular lesson. The children explore these action words while on the run. Call the words out using a naturally expressive and dramatic tone of voice. Children respond to enthusiasm and love to repeat actions. Feel the rhythm of the class to sense how long to stay with a particular exploration. Allow children to explore the action words with isolated body parts, their entire bodies and while they travel through space.

It is important to look at a lesson plan as a guide. Always be prepared for the unexpected when working with children. Unforeseen circumstances may cause the children's attention to lapse. Set your lesson plan aside. Spontaneity may be necessary. Have some "back burner" ideas to introduce. For example, be prepared to play a game. Movement games are contained in the "Game Day" lesson located in Chapter 16.

Creating a Comfortable Environment

It is the teacher's responsibility to create a friendly, respectful and non-competitive environment. The result is a playful and fun atmosphere that instills the love of movement into a child's world. It is important to see every child. Clearly verbalize what a specific child is doing using the movement vocabulary from that lesson. All children want to be an integral part of an activity. Use a child's name and give them a chance to be noticed. In Creative Dance the movements are never imposed upon a child. This creates a nurturing atmosphere of encouragement and acceptance. The steps are not taught. Children are given ample opportunities to feel what it is like to do a step or a movement. A child is never singled out when he doesn't grasp a step. Everyone explores movement together, yet in their own individual way.

It is necessary to keep the dance floor clean and free of obstacles. In a classroom environment, have children help you move aside the desks and chairs. There is an advantage to dancing in a classroom. Children are surrounded by their work from other curricula. The dance room in the school may also be a multipurpose room or a gymnasium. If your environment permits, it is best to allow children to remove their shoes and socks. Dance is definitely a barefoot experience. When barefoot, children feel the weight of their bodies shift and balance.

Preparation and Setting the Ground Rules

Prepare children by setting guidelines for the dance experience. Ask children to use the bathroom and get a drink of water before dance class. Go over safety issues in your classroom. Children should also not chew gum while moving.

No musical accompaniment is necessary for movement improvisation. However, you may choose to have music playing in the background. Keep the volume low to stimulate, yet not interrupt, individual explorations.

Sometimes a prop is introduced to further enhance a child's understanding of movement concepts. You may choose to provide these props or make them with the children.

Dance is definitely not a regimented experience. Children will get excited and there will be noise. Nevertheless, everyone also pays attention to the action words. Emphasize that dance is a way of talking through movement. Most of the time children will move without talking. There will also be opportunities to accompany movement with voice. You can put both of your arms in the air, which is the signal for "all quiet." Ask children to "throw their voices out the window."

Begin each lesson in a circle. Talk briefly about the elements of movement that will be taught during that lesson.

It is important to designate times for children to express how they feel about a lesson. For example, before each Good-Bye Dance have children sit in a circle. Ask them to verbalize what elements of movement they explored during that lesson. These are elements they will use to invent their own final dances.

Background Information on Joseph Pilates and Rudolf Laban

Joseph Pilates (1880-1967), the originator of the Pilates method of exercise, was a fitness trainer as well as a circus performer. His New York City Pilates studio was established in 1926 when he arrived from Europe. It attracted such innovative modern dancers as Martha Graham and ballet master George Balanchine. Emphasizing his multidisciplined approach, Pilates worked extensively with dancers to improve their level of performance or to rehabilitate them from injury.

His fitness program was an amalgamation of many different disciplines that he had studied and practiced. These included ballet, yoga, the martial arts and physical therapy. The Pilates method of exercise emphasizes the principles of movement present in all of these disciplines. In this Creative Movement program, children receive an original introduction to these essential "ABC" principles of movement. **Alignment, breathing** and **centering** are a delightful way to enhance the exhilarating kinesthetic moments within Creative Movement.

The
ABC
Principles of Movement:

• Alignment

• Breathing

• Centering

Before coming to America, Joseph Pilates worked with European pioneers of dance, including Rudolf Laban. **Rudolf Laban** (1879-1958) was an architect, dancer and movement theorist who founded the clear language of the elements of movement. He referred to them as **time, space, effort, shape** and **flow**. Every time we move, we use each of these elements of movement. Children creatively explore these Laban-based elements of movement in this program. They improvise ways of moving and structure dances in response to these action words.

Laban's theories of the body and its relationship to effort and space have influenced such fields as architecture, dance, sports, fitness, movement therapy, physical rehabilitation, psychology, corporate management and Creative Dance for children.

Laban participated in the major European artistic activities of his time, including the development of modern dance. He also created Labanotation—an intricate notation system for movement, much like the notation of music. It is used primarily to record dance choreography.

Chapter 1

Warm Up with the ABC Exercises

The ABC exercises are like vitamin supplements, boosting your immune system and helping children and you feel great!

These are non-competitive, "internal" warm-up exercises. You will immediately see children's concentration, relaxation and strength improve.

What are the ABCs?

- **Alignment** exercises line up the bones and help make it easier for joints and muscles to move.

- **Breathing** exercises nourish the muscles.

- **Centering** core stomach muscle contractions replenishes organs.

How do they help?

- They help students feel calm.

- They improve kids' ability to concentrate on their schoolwork.

- They help children relax after being in a stressful situation, such as an argument with a sibling.

- They help when children are sick.

Putting the ABCs into everyday use:

- When it gets close to lunchtime and the class gets "wiggly," stop for a moment. Spending just a few minutes with the ABC exercises will help children breathe deeply and make them calm and more focused.

- By incorporating movement into the lesson, kids will have a broader understanding of the subject. The ABC exercises let you discuss the skeleton (**The As: alignment**), the respiratory system (**The Bs: breathing**) and the muscles (**The Cs: centering abdominal movements**).

How do the ABCs work to create a lifetime of healthy habits?

Alignment, Breathing and Centering are elements that are not only essential for every efficient dance, sport and fitness movement, they are also some of the key ingredients for increasing your energy level. This can lead to an acceleration of the body's natural healing process after an injury or illness. The same ABCs that help a dancer appear to be floating can be used to help elevate your energy to re-establish body harmony.

You can build your energy level through **Breathing** and/or involving your core abdominal muscles. This is accomplished by giving your respiratory system and internal organs additional blood and oxygen!

The **Breathing** exercise balances and calms your nervous system. The **Centering** exercise strengthens your deep abdominal muscles. This core strength provides you with great posture, back support, internal organ health and efficiency of motion. Plug the powerful **Centering** exercise directly into any sport, martial art, dance or fitness movement to get the following benefits:

1. Safety
2. Play at your best "in the zone."
3. Boost your immune system.

These healing tools are helpful not only when the body is stressed or out of balance. They can be done anytime, anywhere and in any position—standing in the lunch line, sitting at your desk or waiting for the bus!

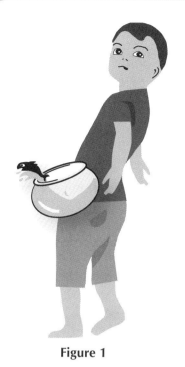

Figure 1

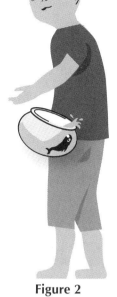

Figure 2

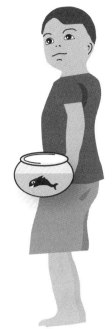

Figure 3

A is for *Alignment*:
The Pelvis as a Fish Bowl Exercise™

1. Begin by standing. Pull your stomach muscles inward toward your spine. Visualize your navel moving toward your spine.

2. Picture your pelvis as a fish bowl.

3. The rim of the fish bowl is your waistline. Place your hands on your waist to feel the top of your fish bowl.

4. Slightly tip your hips forward. Visualize water dumping out of the top of your fish bowl in front of you. The lower back arches. (Figure 1)

5. Tilt your fish bowl backwards. Slosh water on the floor behind you. The lower back rounds. (Figure 2)

6. Now balance your pelvis as a fish bowl. Not a drop of water spills. (Figure 3) You have a slight "natural curve" in your lower back. Tightening your stomach muscles, too, helps keep the fish in the bowl.

7. Keep your fish bowl level while you stand up, walk and sit down. Try it! Did the fish fall out when you were standing, walking or sitting?

8. Tighten your abdominal muscles while performing Pelvis as a Fish Bowl. Try the exercise again while standing up, walking and sitting down. Notice that by contracting your abdominal muscles you take the pressure off your knees, hip joints, back and neck. The weight of your body lifts upward from your legs and away from the floor. You are moving through space from your center abdominal muscles like a martial artist!

> **Float in the air!**
> When you contract your abdominal muscles, you take the pressure off your knees, hip joints, back and neck. The weight of your body lifts upward from your legs and away from the floor!

B is for *Breathing*:

The Three-Dimensional Breathing Exercise™

We'll do this exercise standing, but it can be done anytime, in any position!

Remember, these are deep, slow, even and tranquil inhalations and exhalations.

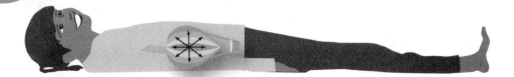

Start

1. Let your inhalations make your body feel tall, wide and thick.

2. Picture a long, wide and thick balloon inside your body. Visualize filling this balloon with air from top to bottom, side to side and across your body. *Try this several times.*

3. Inhale and imagine your body stretching from the inside outward. See your balloon expand to have length, width and depth. Remember, this happens on your long and slow inhalation.

4. Exhale and picture the balloon in your mind's eye shrinking from all three directions. Remember that your balloon deflates into the center of your body on your slow exhalations.

5. *Take several long, slow and tranquil breaths.*

6. Inhale and envision your body as a hot air balloon that you are inflating. Exhale and watch the hot air balloon collapse. Alternate filling your hot air balloon vertically (top to bottom), then horizontally (side to side) and finally sagitally (crossways) during a **single inhalation**. Exhale. (Figure 4)

7. Try mixing up the directions of your single inhalation between length, width and depth. Clearly picture each separate direction in your mind while inhaling. While practicing a single inhalation, say to yourself, "Up and down, then side-to-side and finally forward and backwards." Exhale.

C is for *Centering* (Core Abdominal Control)
The Foundation Exercise™ at a Glance

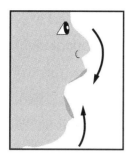

Step 1: Contract your stomach muscles like a **JAW** clamping shut within your trunk.

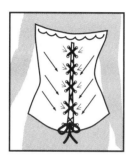

Step 2: Contract your stomach muscles like a **CORSET** cinching your rib cage together and downward.

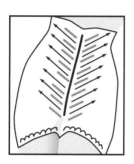

Step 3: Contract your stomach muscles like a **GIRDLE** tightening inwards, backwards and upwards.

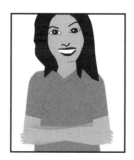

Step 4: Contract your stomach muscles like an internal **HUG** wrapping around the body.

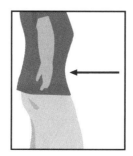

Step 5: Contract your stomach muscles as if sinking your **NAVEL** in toward your spine.

Play with Your Breathing to Tighten Your Tummy

Allow children to practice one step at a time several times in a row to really feel their abdominal muscles contract. For example, tell them to contract the abdominals while imagining the motion of a **jaw closing** along the front of their trunk . . . inhale keeping the muscles tightened, exhale to close the jaw together tighter. **Exhale** forcefully to help contract the deep abdominal muscles. Then **inhale** while maintaining the abdominal contraction. Whether taking air in or letting it out, the abdominals should **never relax**.

The Foundation Exercise™: Breaking Down the Steps

Why learn the Foundation Exercise™?

This exercise is the key to successfully performing challenging activities or sports, or even something as simple as properly lifting a heavy object.

How it helps:

- This is a great exercise to do before recess, physical education or sports.

- You can teach the children to do the Foundation Exercise™ before they swing a bat, a tennis racket or a golf club. The result? A more even, powerful swing that uses ALL their strength.

- Before your karate kick, tighten your stomach muscles like a jaw clamping shut. WOW! You get even more power!

Position for the Foundation Exercise™: Standing

(But it can be performed in any position.)

Start the Foundation Exercise™

Exercise continues on the following page.

Step 1:

Picture a jaw closing within your tummy.

- Inhale fully.

- Lengthen the sound of your exhale as you contract your abdominals, like a **jaw** clamping shut inside your trunk. This feels like your ribs and hips come together at your waistline.

Imagine . . .
Your tummy pulling together like a **jaw** closing.

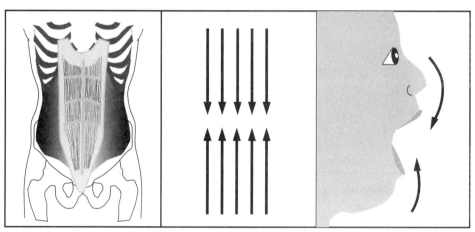

Rectus Abdominis	**Direction of muscle fibers and contraction**	**Imagine for abdominal contraction: jaw closing**

This is the outermost layer of your abdominals. The muscle fibers run vertically. They originate at the pubic bone and insert beneath the breastbone.

Keep your abdominals tight while you inhale. Continue with Step 2 . . .

Step 2:

Picture cinching a corset around your rib cage.

• Exhale powerfully as you contract your stomach muscles like a **corset** cinching your ribs together in the front of your body.

Imagine . . .
Your tummy is like the strings of a **corset**—pulling in and down.

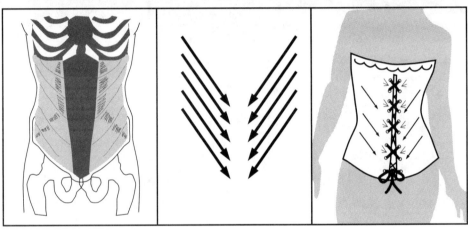

| External Obliques | Direction of muscle fibers and contraction | Imagine for abdominal contraction: corset |

This is the second layer of your abdominals. The muscle fibers run in diagonal slants. They originate at the lower eight ribs and insert at the top of the pelvis.

Keep your abdominals tight while you inhale. Continue with Step 3 . . .

Step 3:

Picture the powerful elastic action of a girdle tightening your abdominal wall in, back and up.

• Exhale forcefully and contract your stomach muscles like a **girdle** that pulls your hip area in, back and up.

Imagine . . .
Your tummy pulling together like a **girdle** in, back and up.

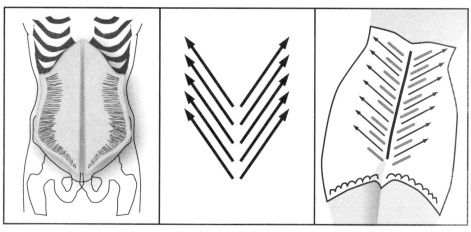

| **Internal Obliques** | **Direction of muscle fibers and contraction** | **Imagine for abdominal contraction: girdle** |

This is the third layer of the abdominals. The muscle fibers run in diagonal slants. They originate at the pelvic rim and insert on the last four ribs.

Keep your abdominals tight while you inhale. Continue with Step 4 . . .

Step 4:

Picture an internal hugging motion deep inside your tummy.

- Exhale strongly as you activate your stomach muscles like an internal **hug** wrapping around the body.

Imagine . . .
Your tummy coming together like a seat belt being pulled across your stomach. This feels like a strong **hug** inside your tummy.

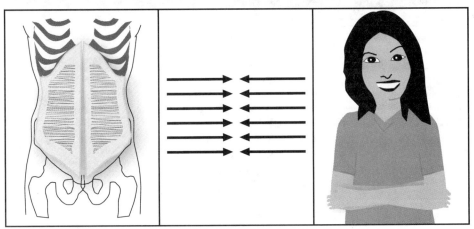

| Transverse Abdominis | Direction of muscle fibers and contraction | Imagine for abdominal contraction: hug |

This is the fourth and deepest layer of your abdominals. The muscle fibers run horizontally. They originate at the pelvic rim and the cartilage of the last six ribs. They insert at the breastbone and pubic bone.

Keep your abdominals tight while you inhale. Continue with Step 5 . . .

Step 5:

Picture sinking your navel in far enough for it to rest on your backbone.

- Exhale as you contract your abdominal muscles as if you are sinking your **navel** into your spine.

Imagine . . .

Your belly button is sinking inward toward your spine.

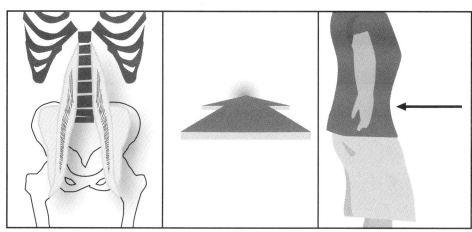

| **Iliopsoas** | **Arcs toward spine and direction of contraction** | **Imagine for abdominal contraction: navel to spine** |

You have finished the Foundation Exercise™!

The Science Behind the Foundation Exercise™

Pilates was designed to train the deeper functional muscles of the body. This emphasis on the smaller, postural muscles provides support for the larger, superficial structural muscles of the body. *Functional Fitness* training is fitness from the inside out. The Foundation Exercise™ helps you activate deeper layers of the abdominal muscles which are responsible for proper breathing, good posture and organ and spine support.

It is helpful to first picture the abdominals to find them, and then feel them contract. The abdominal muscles are made up of four layers of powerful elastic bands.

These abdominal muscles crisscross to form an anatomical girdle. They lie across each other at various angles. (Figure 5)

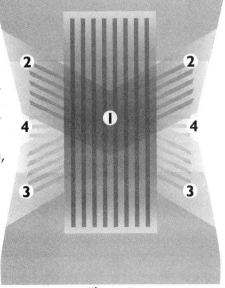

Figure 5

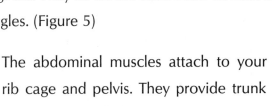

How it helps:
Teach children how to do a sit-up correctly with the Foundation Exercise! Just remember JAW-CORSET-GIRDLE-HUG-NAVEL.

The abdominal muscles attach to your rib cage and pelvis. They provide trunk stability and mobility.

Every Pilates movement emanates from your abdominal muscles. In the Foundation Exercise™, visual imagery and picturing your anatomy are combined to provide a shortcut to feel the deep contraction of your abdominal muscles toward your spine.

This exercise requires concentration. Mastering this centering technique provides success and safety for all of your exercises, sports, dance, martial arts and life.

The Four Abdominal Muscle Groups
These are the abdominal muscles from the outermost layer to the deepest layer within the body.

1. Rectus Abdominis

2. External Obliques

3. Internal Obliques

4. Transverse Abdominis

The abdominal muscles contract as a unit to produce movements. Nevertheless, the **Foundation Exercise™** uses visual imagery to isolate each of the four layers of your abdominal muscle groups, step-by-step.

Picturing the anatomy of the abdominal muscles helps you to tone your stomach area like never before. A strong abdominal core offers limitless reserves of power for any activity, making it possible to reach your full movement potential.

Memorize and repeat to yourself, "JAW, CORSET, GIRDLE, HUG, NAVEL."

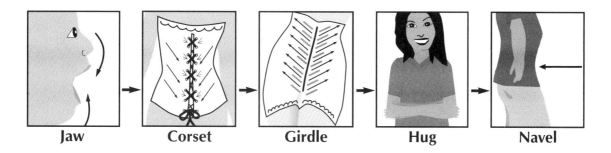

| Jaw | Corset | Girdle | Hug | Navel |

Let the children repeat the five steps of the **Foundation Exercise™** often. It will become a healthy fitness habit for a lifetime!

Reminder:

- The abdominals contract during the exhalation.
- The belly stays tight during the inhalation.
- Try breathing into the back of the ribs, not the belly. This way the four layers of the abdominal muscles contract deeper and deeper toward the spine.

Chapter 2

Laying the Groundwork

Preparation

Place small X shapes on the floor using tape. Leave plenty of space between each X.

This lesson introduces the following:

- Name Rhythms
- Room and Spatial Orientation
- Your Own "Self-Space"
- Locomotor movements while staying in place
- Body Parts on Your "Self-Space"
- The importance of Movement and Stillness

Name Rhythms

Begin by sitting in a circle on the floor. The circle provides a friendly, close gathering. Introduce each child. Then ask the group to clap as they repeat a child's name several times. This is an opportunity for each child to be recognized individually, while simultaneously being part of a group.

"Name Rhythms" is a wonderful rhythmic activity. It not only helps children maintain a basic pulse beat, but also helps them to learn where to place the appropriate accents. You can develop this further in future lessons by utilizing musical instruments. Children can even make their own instruments or create them from household items.

Start the Lesson

Room and Spatial Orientation

Children will become familiar with the room in which they will be dancing (its floor, walls, ceiling, etc.) as you call out the following directions:

1. Stretch . . . stretch . . . stretch your elbows while moving to the window.

2. Shake your stomach as you travel to the door.

3. Lead with your back while moving to the chalkboard.

Repeat this many times, changing body parts and room destinations. You can ask the children to decide what body part to emphasize, how to move it and where to go with it.

Explore Your Own "Self-Space"

Self-Space means "the space occupied by a single child." It also refers to the area a child can reach in all the directions around his or her own body. It includes sitting, standing and lying down shapes that stay in one place in space.

Find your own X on the floor. This is your "Self-Space." Your "Self-Space" is the area you can reach in all directions around your body without touching a classmate. Reach into all the space around your body while staying on your X.

Call out locomotor movements to perform on the X. For example:

- Jump on your spot.
- Run in place as fast as you can.
- Run slowly on the X.
- Find different ways to leap over your spot.
- Turn and twist on your X.

- Try turns and spins on high, medium and low levels.
- Hop on your spot changing legs.
- Hop over your spot in different ways.

Repeat each of these actions several times.

Body Parts on Your "Self-Space"

One at a time, place your hand, bottom, back, belly, toes, elbows, arms and top of the head on your "Self-Space" while stretching the rest of your body away.

For example, place your hand on the X. Stretch the rest of your body away from your hand.

- Put your foot on your X. Then find a way to stretch your foot as far away from your X as you can. Try this same activity with your ear, arm, belly, hand, back, etc. This involves putting a single body part on the spot, and then reaching it away from the spot.

- Lead with one part of your body all over your "Self-Space." Don't move away from it. For example, move your elbow around, over and across your X.

- Circle your elbow above, behind and below you while using your entire body to change levels from high and low. Repeat this calling out different body parts to circle on high and low levels.

- Find several exciting ways to surround your X. Use your body to make upside-down shapes. For example, balance on your hands and feet with your bottom in the air. What would happen if you lifted one leg in that position?

- Can you balance on your hands and feet with your belly facing the ceiling?

Movement and Stillness

It is important that children understand that creating stillness, or a frozen shape, requires tension. For example, tell the children to use all of their muscles to hold a shape. When the signal to "freeze" is given, the child remains immobile in the shape of that particular moment.

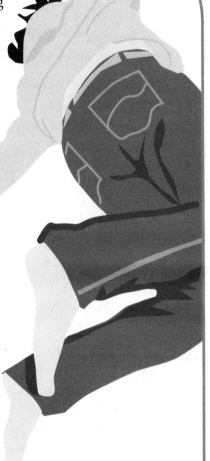

Jump on your spot, turn and twist and try spins on high, medium and low levels.

Repeat the following activities several times:

- Move very quickly and then freeze suddenly into stillness—do not even move an eyelash. Repeat several times changing the amount of time they move and hold a shape.

- Shake your whole body as fast as you can and then freeze it. Hold that shape while I take a picture with an imaginary camera.

- Move as slowly as you can and then freeze like a statue.

- Explore curled, wide and gnarled statue shapes. Add frozen moments. Use your muscles to hold your statue still.

Good-Bye Dance for Laying the Groundwork Lesson

Have children sit in a circle before each Good-Bye Dance. Talk about what you explored during class. This is a time for children to briefly discuss their movement experience.

The child invents his or her own movements during this final dance. The teacher may assist by suggesting elements of movement explored during that class.

Divide the class in half. The children can either perform or watch the other dancers perform. Each group gets a turn.

Start the Good-Bye Dance

- **Find your own X. Freeze in any starting shape on your X.** You may choose to call out some of the shapes from class. For example, freeze in a bent, wide, flat or round shape.

- **Move away from your X any way you wish.** You may suggest running, jumping, walking and turning as the children travel throughout the room. Carry your "Self-Space" with you. Encourage movement into the empty spaces away from other students.

- **Return to your X. Freeze in any final shape that you choose.**

Elements
of Movement: Space
Pathways: Curvy, Straight
and Zigzag
Levels: High/Medium/Low
Shape: Wide/Narrow

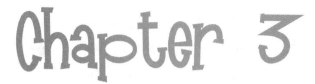

Explore the Basics

Preparation
Place small X shapes on the floor. Leave plenty of space between the Xs.

Start the Lesson
Trace straight and curvy lines while on your "Self-Space."

Entire Body
The group sits in a large circle. Everyone takes an imaginary piece of chalk out of the air.

Trace straight lines above, below, behind and in front of you. Give the children time to explore each area in space around their bodies. Try small and large movements.

Make lots of curvy lines above, below, behind and in front of you. Trace curvy lines above you and freeze in a round shape. Begin to trace curvy lines again, and then freeze in another circular shape. Ask the children to trace several circles. At different intervals, ask students to form the shape of a circle with their bodies and then freeze.

The Zip, Chucka, Dot Dance
Non-Locomotor Movements Using the Entire Body
Everyone will make the following sounds while tracing imaginary lines in the space around them.

- Say "Zip" repetitively while moving your body from a low level to a high level.

The children will use their fingers to trace several straight lines in front of their body while also changing levels. Try explosive jumps from a crouched position. *Repeat this activity several times.*

- Say "Chucka, chucka, chucka" while gradually moving your body downward from a high level to a low level. Rise again. Trace lots of sharp, angular lines in the space in front of your body. *Repeat these percussive movements many times.*

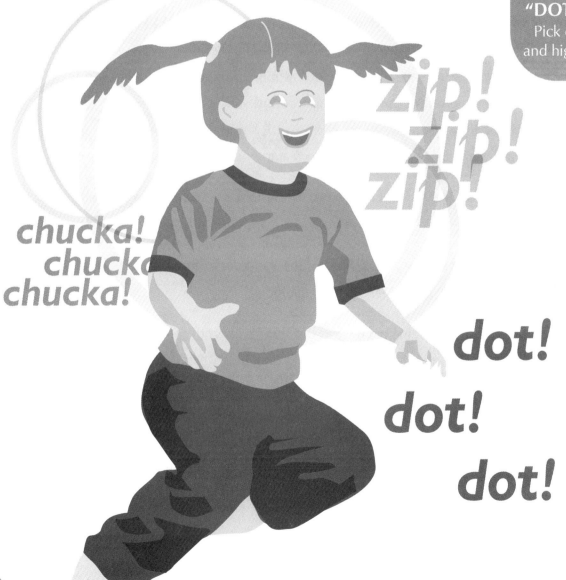

"ZIP!"
Move from a low level to a high level.

"CHUCKA, CHUCKA, CHUCKA!"
Move from a high level to a low level.

"DOT, DOT, DOT!"
Pick out low, medium and high spots in the air.

zip! zip! zip!

chucka! chucka chucka!

dot! dot! dot!

- Say "Dot, dot, dot," for designating different spots in space on low, medium and high levels. This is like putting periods or exclamation points in the air. Gradually increase the rhythm.

Make a sequence of movements. Repeat the combination several times. For example, "zip" while moving the body upward, "chucka, chucka, chucka" while moving downward and "dot, dot, dot" while moving on low, medium and high levels. Use the words as an accompaniment to the varied rhythm.

Try placing the dots in front of you, to your right side, to your left side, behind, above and below you.

Locomotor Steps While Traveling in Curvy, Zigzag and Straight Pathways

Skip, walk, run, gallop and slide throughout the room. Periodically ask students to stop and freeze in either a round or a straight shape. For example: skip throughout the room and now freeze in a round shape. *Repeat each activity several times.* Skip while weaving in and out among your classmates and freeze in a straight shape, then skip again making quick changes of direction.

- Run in curvy and/or straight pathways throughout the room. Also try walks, gallops, skips, jumps and slides in curvy and straight pathways.

- Use your finger to draw zigzag lines in the space in front of you. These are very sharp, angular lines. Make them gigantic.

- Trace small and large zigzag lines on the floor with your feet while walking or running. Be very precise when changing directions. You may even have to run in place or make quick stops.

- Use your finger to trace small and big curvy lines in the space in front of you.

- Walk, run, skip and slide while tracing small and gigantic curvy lines on the floor.

The EE . . . OO . . . AA Dance:

Non-Locomotor Movements Exploring Wide and Narrow Shapes Using the Entire Body

• Find an X on the floor.

• Make narrow, wide and bent shapes on a high level in space. Accompany these high shapes with the sound "EE."

• Try making wide shapes on a medium level in space. Accompany your shapes with the sound "OO." For example, stretch forward, backwards, sideways and balance on one leg.

• Make round and flat shapes on a low level in space. Accompany your shapes by making an "AA" sound.

• Combine the different levels in space. Try a high stretch on "EE," a wide stretch on "OO" and a low bend on "AA." Repeat several times, changing the rhythm from fast to slow and slow to fast.

> **"EE . . ."**
> Explore shapes on a high level in space.
>
> **"OO . . ."**
> Explore shapes on a medium level in space.
>
> **"AA . . ."**
> Explore shapes on a low level in space.

Good-Bye Dance

The group sits in a circle. Ask children what they worked on today. Divide the class in half. One group performs their final dance while the others watch. Give each group a turn.

Start the Good-Bye Dance

• Start in any frozen shape you choose on your spot.
• Go for a journey away from your spot in straight, curvy or zigzag pathways. Find a way to return to your spot.
• Freeze in a shape on your spot.

Call out the action words explored during the lesson. For example: run, slide, skip and gallop in straight, curvy and zigzag pathways. Try bent, wide, flat, round and pointed shapes.

Elements of Movement: Space

Levels:
High/Medium/Low

Directions: Forward/
Backwards/Right Side/
Left Side

Chapter 4

Locomotor Movements

Children explore the basic locomotor steps: walk, run, skip, jump, hop, gallop and slide. Encourage the children to watch for empty spaces when moving about the room. Ask them to dart into the open spaces where there are no other classmates. Explain that dancers and athletes enjoy moving into empty space with quick changes of direction, and the ability to stop quickly. Instruct each child to "carry his or her Self-Space" when moving throughout the dance space.

Start the Lesson

Locomotor Steps Leading with Body Parts

• The group begins sitting in a circle.

• Look up, down, to the right, to the left, behind you, at your neighbor, into the circle and away from the circle.

• Imagine you can put eyes on your nose. Rise, and run throughout the room while leading with your nose.

• Try to move around the room letting one part of your body lead the movement. Change by leading with a different part of your body.

For example:

- **Skip** high leading with your knees.

- **Jump** leading with the top of your head.

- **Slide** leading from your hips.

- Can you change the direction of your **slides**? Slide forward, backwards and sideways.

- **Run** through the space leading with your chest.

- **Run** in place.

- **Run** backwards leading from your bottom.

- Keep **turning** while leading with your elbows.

- Try **walking** very low while making sharp changes of direction. Lead from your feet.

Repeat these activities several times.

Locomotor Steps

Begin at one end of the room. Move to the other side of the room. Perform each of the following locomotor steps many times:

Run, walk, skip, jump, gallop, hop, slide, leap, giant steps, tiptoe and roll to the other side of the room.

Use all of the space to explore each of the following steps:

Perform a high walk, silly walk, stiff march, bouncy walk, floating, stargazing, heavy walk, jerky walk, slow-motion walk, stroll, shaky walk, hobble, backwards walk, sideways walk, curvy walk and straight walk.

Give students plenty of time to fully explore each of these movements.

Invent New Locomotor Steps

Try a cross-legged walk, duck walk, heel-slapping walk, straight-legged walk, knee lifts, bear walk, jumping jacks, inchworms, rabbit jumps and crab walks. Crab walks are performed on your hands and feet with your belly facing the ceiling.

Good-Bye Dance

The group sits in a circle. What did we work on today? Divide the class in half. Give each group a turn.

Start the Good-Bye Dance
- Freeze in any starting shape you choose.
- Invent a new step. Travel throughout the room with this new step.
- Bring your dance to a close. Find an interesting ending shape.
- Freeze in the shape.

Ask each child to give his or her new step a name. Write the name on the chalkboard. If time permits, you may want to end the class by having students briefly try each new step. The choreographer shows the group their new step. Give each child a turn.

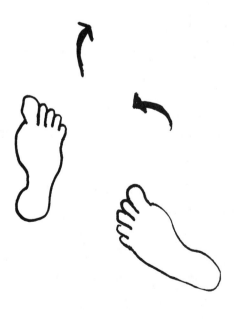

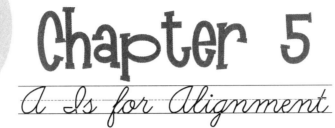

Principle of Movement: Alignment

Elements of Movement: Free Flow/Loose and Bound Flow

Kinetics: Gravity, The Body, Energy

Chapter 5
A Is for Alignment

Bones

This lesson emphasizes movement initiation from the joints and their inherent movement possibilities. These are jazz-dance-like movements. They include movement isolations, joint articulation and sequential mobility of the spine. The joints and bony segments of the body facilitate the following movements: flexion, extension, abduction (limb moves away from the midline of the body), adduction (limb moves in toward the midline of the body), circumduction (circling) and internal and external rotation. Exploring joint mobility produces either efficient free-flow movements or angular bound-flow movements. For example, there is the loose-limbed Scarecrow and the rigid Tin Man in *The Wizard of Oz.*

You may want to teach the names of the bones to the children. An actual skeleton or picture of one is a helpful visual aide. This could also be used as a fun Halloween lesson.

We're going to dance without our muscles today! Try to imagine that we're only made up of bones and joints.

Start the Lesson
Body Parts

• Start by sitting in a circle, Make sure there is plenty of room between one another.

• Move and circle your finger bones, wrist bones, elbows, arm bones, shoulders, shoulder blades, breast bone, rib cage, spine, neck, middle back, lower back, jaw, eyes, forehead, nose, hip bones, knees, legs, ankles, feet and toes. *Repeat this several times.*

• Experiment with all the ways your joints move.

Entire Body

- Focus on using your bones, not your muscles. How many different ways can you twist, bend, stretch and turn your whole body? For example, continuously change your twisting shapes while moving on high and low levels.

Locomotor Movements Using Your Bones

- Go across the room. Move without focusing on your muscles. Try to use just your bones and joints. Your muscles will stay supple and relaxed.

- Come back with "floppy bones."

- How many different things can you do with your bones while moving from one end of the room to the other? Try shaking, hobbling, dragging, melting, spinning, rolling, rising, shuffling, prancing, tiptoeing, marching, kicking, leaping, whipping and flinging your bones. *Repeat several times, adding direction changes.* For example, shake your bones while traveling backwards and sideways.

- Move fast/slow and high/low while rattling and creaking your bones.

- Take your skeleton for a jog, skip, jump, gallop and slide.

Skeleton Dance

- The group sits in a circle. What did we explore today?

- Find a spot out on the dance floor. Choose your own starting shape using your bones. Freeze it.

- When the clock strikes midnight, the skeletons rise.

- Do a fantastic dance using your bones.

- Return to your dwelling while rattling your bones, or return as lazy bones.

- Freeze in a skeleton shape.

Good-Bye Monster Dance in Costume

Preparation

Make a monster costume by crumpling up pieces of paper. Each child puts a few pieces of paper inside his clothing. This changes the shape of their body. Now ask the children to use their muscles to dance.

- Divide the class in half. Give each group a turn to perform.

Start the Good-Bye Dance

- Start frozen in a mean, nice, old or young monster-like shape.
- Make gigantic/tiny, strong/weak, fast/slow and twisted/straight movements. *Repeat several times.* Let each child find many monster shapes.
- Take your monster for a run, hobble, skip and gallop.
- Find a way to bring your journey to a close. Freeze in a final shape.

What's your favorite monster?

Is it big or little?
Strong or weak?
Fast or slow?

Skeleton Dance Summary

- Freeze in a starting shape.
- Rise.
- Fantastic skeleton dance.
- Return with rattling or lazy bones.
- Freeze in a skeleton shape.

Good-Bye Monster Dance Summary

- Freeze in a mean, nice, old, or young monster shape.
- Giant/tiny, strong/weak, fast/slow and twisted/straight movements.
- Run, hobble, skip and gallop.
- Freeze in a final shape.

Chapter 6

Buildings, Subways and Drawbridges

Start the Lesson

Explore Big and Little Locomotor Steps

Students will begin by altering the amount of space they move in. The range is either very small or big.

Repeat the following directions on pages 50-51 several times. Vary the time given to each activity.

Running

Tiny runs staying in place on your "Self-Space."

Run without traveling very much.

Run covering a lot of space.

Skipping

Tiny skips.

Wide skips covering a lot of space.

Galloping

Gallop on your "Self-Space."

Make your gallops bigger and bigger.

Freeze in a wide, stretched-out shape.

Jumping

Small jumps in place.

Tiny jumps that travel.

Big, wide and springy jumps into space.

Tiptoe Steps

Tiny steps on your tiptoes.

Wide steps on your tiptoes.

Slides

Tiny slides.

Big slides.

Ask the class to join hands while making a big circle. Point out the empty space in the center of the circle. This unoccupied area is referred to as "negative space." Tell the class to use their bodies to fill the "positive space."

Large and Small Subway Tunnels Using Body Parts and the Entire Body

Subways often travel through tunnels. Make the shape of a tunnel. Use your body to surround a round shape.

Use different body parts to make small and large tunnels. For example, you can make tunnels with your hands, arms, legs and trunk. Use your entire body to make tunnels. Maybe tiny shapes will surprise you and grow bigger.

Round and Pointed Buildings Using the Entire Body

Make buildings with your entire body. Construct tall, thin, wide, round and pointed buildings using your body. Move the buildings through the space.

Drawbridges Using the Entire Body

The body makes a bridge. Parts of the body are supported on the floor. The rest of the body curves into an arc. Find ways to open the drawbridge.

Frame the space. Use your body to make the shape of a bridge.

Open the drawbridge by lifting different body parts. Try making several different kinds of bridges.

Good-Bye Dance for Buildings, Subways and Drawbridges Lesson

The group sits in a circle. What did we work on today? Divide the class in half.

Preparation

• The teacher picks half of the children to make drawbridges or subway tunnels.

• The other half of the class moves among the drawbridges and tunnels.

Start the Good-Bye Dance

• One group freezes in a bridge or tunnel shape. Keep changing your bridge and tunnel shapes.

• The other group finds different ways to move around the shapes. Try running, slithering or using cross-legged steps. Can you discover ways to put body parts or your entire body into a tunnel? Move under or over a bridge.

• Switch groups. Give each group a chance to experience either making shapes or traveling over, around and through them.

Props:
Beanbags and Rocks
Elements of Movement:

Force: Heavy/Light
Kinetics: Controlled Momentum, Balance and Weight Shifts

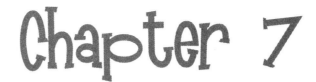

Chapter 7

Beanbags and Rocks

Preparation

- Visit hobby, fabric and craft stores. They have beanbags and small, smooth, multi-colored rocks that can be used for this activity.

- Pass out the beanbags and rocks. Let each child feel them. Shake the beanbags.

- Collect these props for now.

Start the Lesson

Body Parts, Non-Locomotor Movements and Locomotor Steps—Shaking

- The group sits in a circle. Leave plenty of space between each dancer.

- Ask children to explore the quality of shaking. Shaking can be performed with several body parts as well as the entire body. The following sequences examine the characteristics of shaking:

  - While sitting and standing **shake your fingers, hands, toes, feet, belly, back and entire body like a beanbag**.

  - Call out different body parts to **shake up high, down low, in front and to either side** of the body.

  - Stand and **shake the entire body on a high level. Shake your body on a low level**. Try small shakes while lying down with your toes, ankles, legs, hands and arms.

  - Sit and **shake your arms in big, slow movements** forward, backwards and sideways to the right and left.

  - **Run anywhere in the room.** Turn when you choose while shaking your body.

  - **Jump and twirl** with imaginary beanbags inside you.

Investigate the Smooth Shapes of Rocks

- Can you turn your body into the shape of a round rock? Try small and large rock-like shapes.

- Try smooth, circling movements above, below and behind you using your upper body. Imagine you are tracing the shapes of the rocks.

- Take your rock shapes for a run. Try changing directions forward and backwards. Show lots of circular pathways on the floor.

- How many ways can you skip, slide, swing, rise and collapse in circular pathways?

Heavy and Light Movements

- Imagine picking up rocks and putting them in an imaginary bucket. Find light, tiny rocks while walking, tiptoeing, turning and running fast. Give children time to try out each step.

- Gather gigantic rocks while dragging, leaning, pushing and pulling them. Allow them to experiment with each of these very different qualities of movement.

- What's happened to your imaginary bucket?
  Drag your heavy bucket behind you.
  Dump the imaginary rocks out of the bucket. Use all of your muscles.
  Repeat this activity several times.

- Shake, shake, shake the rocks out of the bucket.

Beanbag Dance

• Give each child a beanbag.

Body Parts

Using beanbags, explore the following balance and weight shift movements several times:

• Balance the beanbag on your hand, shoulder, head or knee. What would happen if you traveled while balancing the beanbag on various body parts? Give students plenty of time to examine moving and balancing with a prop.

• Move high, low, crouch, turn and tiptoe while balancing the beanbags. Call out each of these directions one at a time. Use your arms to help you balance.

• Balance the beanbag. Travel and collapse when the beanbag falls. Continue moving. Explore rising, balancing and collapsing.

Good-Bye Dance for the Beanbags and Rocks Lesson

- The class sits in a circle. What elements of movement did we examine today?
- Divide the class in half. Give each group a turn to perform.
- In this Good-Bye Dance the teacher calls out directions while the children choose their own solutions.

Start the Good-Bye Dance

Locomotor Movements

Hold the beanbag on different body parts while moving from one end of the room to the other in the following ways:

- Freeze in any starting shape you choose with your beanbag.
- Hold your beanbag against various body parts while you skip, jump, hop, slide, wiggle, shuffle and gallop.

Slide the beanbag along the floor. Move to it in the following ways:

- Scoot, twirl, drag and run in straight and curvy pathways.
- Toss the beanbag in the air. Catch it with a body part. *Repeat this activity several times.*
- Find a challenging shape to freeze in.

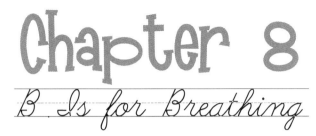

Principle of Movement: Breathing Space

Levels: Free Flow/Loose and Bound Flow

Kinetics: Gravity, The Body, Energy

Chapter 8

B Is for Breathing

Meteorites

For this lesson, you may want each child to make their own meteorites.

Preparation

How to Make a Meteor:

- Take a square piece of aluminum foil. Gather the center together into the shape of a bow tie.

- Use long plastic bread bags. Cut the bags into strips about 2 inches in width and 3½ feet in length. You will have approximately four strips of plastic.

- You can ask the children to help tie the plastic strips around the center of the tinfoil.

- Crumple the foil into a tight ball. The plastic strips are the fiery tail of the meteor. You now have a meteor.

> ### Know Your Meteorites
>
> **Meteor:** Any of the small particles of matter in the solar system, which are directly observable only by their incandescence from frictional heating on entry into the atmosphere. They produce a sudden or temporary brilliance. A meteorite is a meteor that reaches the surface of the earth without being completely vaporized.

When children throw their meteor, the weight of the foil ball carries it through the air. The plastic strands catch the wind and will waver and make noise. Use the meteors to explore the spatial elements of movement—changing high/medium/low levels while rising and collapsing.

Start the Lesson

Principle of Movement: Breathing

- The group sits in a circle. In addition to your muscles, bones, joints and heart, there is something else that determines how you move. What is it? Breathing. When you breathe your body moves a little bit. Everyone take a big breath. Which way did your body move? Did it move up and down, or out and in? Both. During an inhalation, your trunk expands outward/upward. On the exhalation your trunk deflates inward/downward.

Why use props?

Props encourage children to move freely without embarrassment, and in a variety of ways. Children enjoy observing and imitating the similar and different movement qualities of props.

- Briefly have children lie down on their backs. Ask them to place their hands on their stomach and ribs. Notice how your stomach and ribs rise while taking air into your body. Pay attention to how your stomach and ribs collapse toward the floor while letting air out. This is like relaxation breathing in yoga. Now tighten your stomach muscles while letting the air out. This is like breathing during Pilates fitness training.

Breathing

Large and Small Shapes Using the Entire Body

- Move your whole body to exaggerate the wave-like motion of breathing. Now show me with your body only. Too much breathing will make your throat dry.

- Slowly rise to demonstrate taking air in. Make a large shape. Stretch the shape. Let the body expand as far as possible.

- Collapse to express, letting the air out of your body. Make a small shape.

- Move outward to a large shape and inward to a small shape.

Repeat these activities several times.

58

Sigh

These are sustained movements.

Entire Body

• Show me what a sigh would look like using your whole body.

• These are smooth movements that rise and fall.

Body Parts

• Show me a sigh with your elbow, ear, foot or other body part.

Locomotor Steps

• Take your sigh for a walk, skip, run, jump or other movement.

• Sigh in silence or accompany your sighing movements by saying "Oh well" or "Whatever."

Hiccup

These are percussive movements.

Entire Body

• Make tiny, quick, jerky movements that rise and fall.

• The children experiment with tiny rising and collapsing movements.

• Show me your hiccup dance. Use your entire body.

• These are springy jumps on a low, medium and high level.

• Add light turns.

• Hiccup while traveling backwards and sideways.

Body Parts

• Hiccup your shoulder, eye, neck, finger, back or other body part. Do this without verbal accompaniment (no hiccup sounds). Show me with your body parts.

Sneeze

High/Medium/Low Levels

Entire Body

Combine sustained and percussive movements.

- Use different rhythms. "Aaaaaaaaaa"—sustained, smooth and slow rise to a high level. "Choo"—percussive, strong and fast collapse to a low level. *Rise and collapse your body several times.*

- Try a short, fast and strong percussive "aa—choo." Make continuous short, fast and strong movements. Travel through the space while rising and collapsing.

Body Parts

- Feel the sneeze in your spine, arm, leg or other body part. Use a variety of rhythms. *Repeat these motions several times.*

Locomotion

- Let a great, big, huge sneeze take you from one end of the room to the other. *Repeat this several times.*

- Travel backwards with "aaaaaaaaaa" and run forward with "chooooooooo." *Repeat this activity many times.* Ask children to rise and suspend momentarily on a high level, before running forward—hold . . . hold . . . hold . . . and then run forward. Add variety by fully collapsing the body onto the floor before moving backwards again.

Hand Out the Meteors

Briefly talk about what meteors are. You may choose to do this before the movement lesson. Explain how they collapse straight downward.

High/Medium/Low Levels

Entire Body

- Hold your meteor.

- Shake it high and low. Add frozen moments without any movement. Then shake again.

- Circle the meteors high/low, slow/fast. Try this above or behind your body.

- Combine high and low levels in space with long, sustained and short, percussive movements. Make large, slow and smooth movements. Find small, fast and sharp movements.

Locomotion

- Float through space with your meteor flying behind you.

- Try collapsing your upper body.

- Make a sequence of movements with your meteor. Rise . . . jump . . . run . . . turn . . . and collapse in a low shape. *Call out these action words several times.* Give children time to feel this sequence of movements.

- Keep the meteor near you. Throw it up and then imitate its motion with your body.

- Let the meteor soar through space. Go to it. Move like it did—rising and collapsing.

Meteorite Dance

- You may want to use music.

- Begin with the meteor at the opposite end of the room.

- Freeze in any starting shape you choose.

- Move your body like a meteor. Can you show its fiery tails? Move high and low. Rise and collapse your whole body and body parts.

- Arrive at the meteor. Pick it up. Move with it in place. Shake your body.

- Take it for a journey through outer space.

- Find an ending shape. Freeze in that shape.

Empty Suit of Clothes

- Imagine you are an empty suit of clothes. Show me how your suit of clothes can rise and collapse when you fill it with air or let the air out. For example, imagine filling your shoes with air. Continue making a fun sound like an air pump for accompaniment.

- Everyone fill up one piece of clothing at a time.

- Pump up your socks, trousers, belt, shirt, jacket, bow tie, gloves and hat with air.

- Deflate all of the air out of your suit of clothes and collapse.

- Gradually fill up the clothes with swirling air.

- Collapse the suit of clothes. Let all the air out of it.

- Let the suit rise high and wide by pumping air into it.

- Deflate it.

- Pump the air into it. Move fast and jump high.

- Collapse.

Repeat the above activities several times.

The Good-Bye Dance for the Breathing Lesson

The class sits in a circle. Ask students to talk about the elements of movement they explored in this lesson. You may want to accompany them with a drum or use a vocal sound. Divide the class in half. Give each group a turn to perform.

Start the Good-Bye Dance

• Freeze in a starting shape. Pump up your suit of clothes with air.

• Take your suit of clothes for a journey. Move as you wish.

• Deflate your suit of clothes.

• Freeze in your final shape.

Chapter 9

Telling a Story

Preparation

You may want to prepare with a science lesson about the different stages of a butterfly (see box at left).

The Butterfly Life Cycle

1. The butterfly lays her eggs on the underside of a leaf.

2. In a few days to a week, a caterpillar chews a hole in the shell of the egg and climbs out.

3. Caterpillars shed their skin many times as they grow. They then spin a cocoon or silk casing. The caterpillar hangs upside-down in this cocoon.

4. The hanging caterpillar, or chrysalis, is hibernating while going through amazing physiological changes. It is changing into a butterfly.

5. The cocoon bursts and the butterfly crawls out. After about 30 minutes, the wings harden and the butterfly takes its first flight.

6. The miracle of metamorphosis is complete.

Start the Lesson

Explore Large/Small, and Wide/Narrow Shapes

Body Parts

• The group sits in a circle with plenty of room between each participant.

Curl and then stretch like a rubber band using different body parts.

• Stretch a rubber band between the following body parts one at a time: your fingers, hands, wrists, arms, elbows, legs, knees, ankles, heels and toes. Allow time to experiment with reaching out and curling in for each part of the body.

• Curl and then stretch like a rubber band with your arm/leg, neck/back, finger/toe and leg/head.

Entire Body

Curl into the smallest shape possible and then stretch your body in the following ways:

- Shrink into a narrow shape and then reach out to a very wide shape.

- Explore different round/flat, low/wide and bent/high shapes on the repetitions. For example, shrink into a round shape and then reach way out into a wide shape.

Locomotor Movements

- Begin at one end of the room and end at the other side of the room.

- Stretch . . . stretch . . . stretch a gigantic rubber band using your whole body and then travel in the following ways:

- Begin with a gigantic stretch and then run, gallop, jump, skip, twirl, do a floppy walk and make giant steps. Imagine shooting a rubber band. Now show me with your whole body.

Repeat each locomotor movement several times.

Tell a Story with Your Caterpillar Dance

Make the following caterpillar movements:

- Start frozen in an egg-shape.

- Continuously travel while chewing, climbing, slithering, shrugging, wiggling, pointing, dragging, creeping, twisting, melting, spinning and rolling. Allow plenty of time to explore each of these qualities of movement.

- Try many hanging upside-down shapes.

- Surround yourself with your silk cocoon. Turn, twist and spin in your upside-down shapes.

- Freeze in an upside-down shape. Don't move a caterpillar muscle.

Butterfly

Try several of the following shapes and movements:

- Burst, crawl, bend, stretch, float, jump, hop, tiptoe, twist, turn, stargaze, leap, swing, swoop and fly like a butterfly.

- Find a final butterfly shape to freeze in.

Good-Bye Dance for the Tell a Story Lesson

The group sits in a circle. What did we explore today? Divide the class in half. Give each group a turn to perform.

Start the Good-Bye Dance

- Freeze like a caterpillar inside an eggshell.

Offer suggestions for the following caterpillar movements:

- Chew, climb, slither, shrug, wiggle, crawl, hobble, spin and roll.

- Change directions often by moving forward, backwards and sideways. Use different body parts to show us your knobs, bumps, hair and antennae.

- Find different hanging upside-down shapes.

- Twist and spin them to make your silk cocoon.

Butterfly

- Burst, crawl, bend, stretch, float, jump, hop, tiptoe, twist, turn, stargaze, leap, swoop, light jumps and fly like a butterfly.

- Find a final butterfly shape to freeze in.

Chapter 10

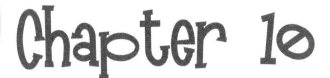

Pathways

Preparation

• Draw curvy and straight lines on the chalkboard.

• You may want to prepare by doing an art project. The children can draw curvy and straight lines.

Start the Lesson

• Begin by spreading out in the room. Students should find their own "Self-Space."

• Take an imaginary piece of paper and a crayon from the air. Trace curvy lines in the air using your crayon.

Body Parts

• Use different body parts to draw curvy lines. For example, trace lots of curvy lines using your hands, arms, back or other body part.

Entire Body

• Make curvy, round shapes with your entire body. Trace curvy lines by swinging, circling, turning, twisting, spinning and rolling your body. Give students time to experience each of these movements.

• Place a piece of imaginary paper in the air. Trace straight lines.

Body Parts

• Use your nose, elbow, back or other body part to draw straight lines in the space around you.

Entire Body

• Make straight, angular shapes with your entire body. Periodically ask them to freeze their bent shapes. *Repeat this several times.*

• Ask everyone to help roll a huge piece of imaginary paper out along the entire floor. Each child travels throughout the entire room.

Locomotor Movements

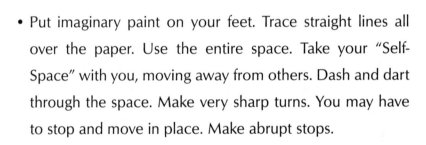

• Begin by finding a bent shape with your body.

• Put imaginary paint on your feet. Trace straight lines all over the paper. Use the entire space. Take your "Self-Space" with you, moving away from others. Dash and dart through the space. Make very sharp turns. You may have to stop and move in place. Make abrupt stops.

• Travel while continuously making razor-like, bent shapes with your whole body.

Vary straight pathways using the following activities, one at a time:

• Run, walk or skip in straight pathways.

• Make sharp changes of direction forward, backwards sideways and turning around corners.

• Freeze in an angular shape.

• Get ready to jump when the the gigantic piece of paper is removed. Everyone help spread out a new sheet of imaginary paper across the floor.

- Find a curvy shape with your body.

- Trace tiny and big, wave-like, curved lines throughout the space around you. What happens when you run in curvy pathways? Your body leans. Lean to the left and right.

- Change directions by moving backwards, sideways and by turning.

- Add curvy shapes to your body while you keep traveling.

- Get ready to jump when the paper is removed. Roll out a new sheet of imaginary paper along the entire floor space.

- Use your body to combine curvy and straight shapes. Maybe your trunk can make a round shape while your knee and elbow bend.

- Move through space tracing curvy and straight pathways.

- Move forward, backwards, sideways and in circles along straight and curvy paths.

- Jump high when the imaginary paper is removed.

Then, trace curvy and straight pathways in each of the following ways: **squish into sand, dash across hot sand, splash through water, sink into mud** and **skitter along the sidewalk** without stepping on the cracks.

While wearing imaginary hiking boots: experiment with **jerky, powerful** and **heavy** qualities of movement. Discover ways to **stagger, drag, chug, pound** and **climb** in your boots.

While wearing imaginary moccasins, try each of the following movements: move **quietly, softly, smoothly, crouching, brushing, fast** and **gently**.

While wearing imaginary cowboy boots, try moving in each of the following cowboy ways: **kicking, galloping, jumping, turning, leaping** and **strutting**.

While wearing flippers for swimming, try moving in each of the following ways: **flicking, sinking, waving, flinging** and **cross-legged steps**.

While wearing pointed elf shoes: move **brightly** and then **sharply**. Try **darting, tapping, wiggling** and performing **tiny jumps**.

Good-Bye Dance for the Pathways Lesson

The group sits in a circle. What did we do today? Give children an opportunity to talk about their experience. Divide the class into two groups. Give each group a turn.

Start the Good-Bye Dance

- Start by wearing imaginary slippers while tracing curvy and straight pathways.

- Freeze in a starting shape.

- What would happen if you moved softly, slowly, tiptoeing? Investigate movements that are heavy and sleepy. What would "fuzzy movements" look like? Move while yawning.

- Freeze in a final curvy or straight shape.

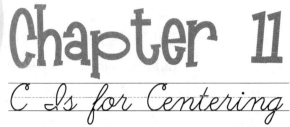

Chapter 11
C Is for Centering

Statues

Preparation

You will need a long piece of tape. Place it on the floor across the center of the room. The children should sit in a circle. Notice as you sit on the floor that your body is making a shape. The sitting shape you are in is different from the person next to you.

Start the Lesson

• On the count of 3, sit in a different shape. Try another shape—1, 2, 3, freeze it. *Repeat several times finding unusual sitting shapes.*

• Try lying down and standing shapes too.

• Tighten your muscles "from the inside." Feel the shape you are in with your deepest muscles. If a blast of air came through, you could hold the shape. This muscular effort is used by martial artists. Martial artists have to remain strong or "centered." That way their opponent can't throw them off balance.

Locomotor Steps and Frozen Shapes

Skip across the room and ➡ freeze in a curled shape.

Jump around the room and ➡ freeze in a high, narrow shape.

Gallop across the room and ➡ end in a wide shape.

Slide and ➡ end in a twisted shape.

Run and ➡ end in a low, flat shape.

Roll and ➡ end in a round ball.

Walk backwards and ➡ end in an upside-down shape.

Repeat the above activities several times.

Freeze and Move the Shape

- Make a tiny shape. Freeze it. Make it move all over the space. Try another small shape. Experiment with round, curled and narrow shapes. Freeze in each shape. Discover ways to travel while maintaining your shape.

- Find many ways to make each of the following shapes. Try out gigantic, puffed up, circular, towering, crouched and wide shapes. Freeze in each shape. Can you find ways to make these shapes while moving around the room?

Repeat the above activities many times.

Flying Shapes

- The class begins on one end of the room. They will run and jump over the tape you placed on the floor.

- Ask students, "What do you know that makes shapes in the air?" Some examples are, a skier going over a jump, a hot air balloon, an ice skater, a kite, an airplane, a bird, a cloud and an astronaut. You may want to have the children make these shapes while going over a jump.

- Divide the class in half and have them take turns.

- Freeze in a starting shape.

- Run and jump over the line of tape.

- Make a stretched out shape while you are in the air. See the guide box for other flying shapes.

- End on the other side of the room in a frozen shape.

Action words to call out for flying shapes:

Turning

Tiny

Gigantic

Narrow

Curvy

Bent

Low

Wide-legged

Twisted

Backwards

Collapsed

Clay

Encourage students not to break out of each shape. Ask them to visualize their body as clay. Try to blend one shape into the next. Keep molding your body into heavy clay shapes like each one of the following:

• Make tiny, round, wide, curvy, straight, twisted and flat shapes.

• Move like heavy clay. Jump, run, slide or gallop like heavy clay.

Wire

• Wire is malleable like clay, but it produces different qualities of movement.

• Move into lots of curvy wire shapes that travel.

Explore each of the following wire shapes:

• Twisting, stretching, spiraling, sharp, straight and corkscrew shapes.

• Take your wire shapes for a run.

• Spring into wire shapes.

• Feel your wire shapes changing into clay shapes. Try doing the opposite.

Repeat these activities several times.

Good-Bye Dance for the Statues Lesson

Sculptors and Statues in Pairs

- The children sit in a circle. Ask them to verbalize what elements of movement they explored in the lesson.

- Prepare the children through a demonstration. The teacher will be the sculptor. Choose a child to be the statue. Gently sculpt the statue into different clay or wire shapes. For example, a light touch on the upper back may make the statue curl forward.

Start the Good-Bye Dance

- Divide the group into pairs.

- Designate who will be the sculptor and who will be the statue.

- Give each child a turn to experience both.

- Children begin to mold their statues into different shapes.

- Guide this final dance by mentioning curvy/straight lines and low/medium/high levels.

- End by asking the sculptors to walk around the statue garden.

- Ask students to use elements of movement as their vocabulary to describe the frozen statues.

Repeat the activity with the "statues" becoming the "sculptors."

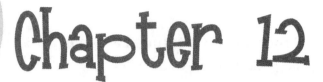

Chapter 12

Pick a Word

In the Pick a Word lesson the children continue to learn the association between verbal and non-verbal communication. They use improvisation to increase their movement vocabulary.

Preparation

You will need to prepare by placing the lesson words on cards. You will have the following two separate decks of cards:

1. Locomotor Steps

Place the words **skip, walk, run, gallop, jump, slide** and **hop** on several cards.

2. Action Words

Place the words **push, big, heavy, zigzag, high, off-balance, prickly, join, soar, halt, sticky, pause, grinning** and **mingle** on several cards.

Start the Lesson

Basic Locomotor Steps: Run, walk, skip, gallop, jump, slide and hop

• Ask each child to choose one locomotor step card. Explore your locomotor step in the following ways:

Level changes—high, medium and low:

Try stepping on high, medium, and low levels.

Directions—forward, backwards and sideways:

Change directions by moving forward, backwards and sideways.

Size—small and large:

Explore tiny steps that barely travel.

Travel through space with gigantic steps.

Speed—fast and slow:

Make very fast steps. Explore moving in slow motion.

Force—light and heavy:

Make steps as light as a feather. Make heavy steps.

Action Words:

push, big, heavy, zigzag, high, off-balance, prickly, join, soar, halt, sticky, pause, grinning and **mingle**

- Each child picks one action word card.

- Give students many opportunities to explore that word. How many ways can you show your action word?

- The entire class explores all of the words. Combine the locomotor steps and the action words. For example, direct children to try variations of all the following action words in combination with running.

Push, big, heavy, zigzag, high, off-balance, prickly, join, soar, stop, sticky, pause, grinning and **mingle**

- For example: run while pushing something heavy.

- Run taking up large amounts of space.

- Show me a heavy run.

- Run in sharp zigzag pathways.

- Try high runs that fall off-balance.

- Explore running with a prickly sensation going up and down your spine.

- Join a classmate while running.

- Run and then find ways to make airborne shapes. Soar through the air like a kite or airplane.

- Run and abruptly stop your forward momentum.

- Run through sticky taffy while pausing several times.

- Mingle with your classmates while grinning.

If time permits, repeat the above directions with the other locomotor steps.

Good-Bye Dance for Pick a Word Lesson

The group sits in a circle. What did we explore today? Have each child pick a locomotor step and an action card. Divide the class in half. One half will become the audience. The other half will be the performers. Ask the audience to figure out the movement words being explored by the performers.

Start the Good-Bye Dance

• Freeze in a beginning shape.

• Move through space using your locomotor step.

• Travel through space exploring your action word.

• Find ways to combine your locomotor step and your action word.

• Freeze in a final shape.

Now the other group should take a turn performing their final dance.

Chapter 13

Places and Environments

Start the Lesson

- Sit in a large circle.

Body Parts

- Curl your toes, fingers, arms or back.

- Stretch each body part.

Rain Puddles

- Imagine there are rain puddles throughout the room.

- Take huge, wide steps over the rain puddles.

- Balance on one leg while moving over the puddles. Let your arms help you to balance.

- Jump into the puddles.

- Hop on the water.

- Shuffle through the water.

- Dash across the puddles.

Mud

Body Parts

- You are stuck in the mud. Name different body parts that are stuck in the mud. Then stretch . . . stretch . . . stretch away using the rest of your body.

Locomotion

- Move heavily through the mud.
- Step high out of the mud while shaking the dirt off of your feet.
- Tiny gallops and stretched-out gallops through the mud.

Marshmallows

Move through the marshmallows in each of the following ways:

- Explore moving smoothly, lightly, spring up, tiptoe, twirl, bounce, float, ooze, collapse, roll and somersault.

- Melt into the marshmallows and rise several times.

On Ice

Move on the ice in each of the following ways:

- Balance on the ice, fall, fast, slow, smooth, slide, soar, push, glide and spin on your bottom or belly.

- Sway and slide from side-to-side, forward and backwards.

Hot Sand

Move across the hot sand in each of the following ways:

- Dance using percussive accents. These are jerky, sharp, jagged and angular movements.

- Squish your toes into the sand.

- Spring, jump, hop and kick your legs up high.

Buzzing Bees

Show me each one of the following movements with your body:

- Move without using your voice. Keep your mouth tightly closed.

- Run as fast as you can with your arms swinging and swatting.

- Dart, swing, shake, swat, wiggle, flick, scratch, stomp, duck, swirl and lean.

- Move low and fast with your mouth tightly closed.

Sleeping Cats

Move among sleeping cats in each of the following ways:

• Creep, crawl, tiptoe, slide and sway.

• Pat and rub the cats.

• Stop quietly while curling and uncurling your body.

• Take wide, soft steps around and over the cats.

Pit Full of Snakes

• Move cautiously around the snakes on low, medium and high levels.

• Bravely run, dodge, jump and leap over the snakes.

• Make twisted, tiny and flat shapes while traveling in curvy paths.

• Travel backwards while looking over your shoulder.

Good-Bye Dance for the Places and Environments Lesson

The group sits in a circle. What did we explore today?

• Divide the room in half. Half of the room contains sleeping cats. The other half is full of buzzing bees.

• Separate the class into two groups. Give each group a turn to perform.

Start the Good-Bye Dance

• Freeze in a starting shape among the bees or cats.

• Move the way you wish through either environment or both.

• Freeze in a final shape.

Chapter 14

Arithmetic

Preparation

Prepare by putting numbers on the floor using tape. Place the numbers far apart from each other.

Start the Lesson

• Go to a number on the floor.

• Place your hands, elbow or ear on the number. Stretch the rest of your body away from it.

• Numbers have curved and/or straight lines.

Body Parts

• Use your finger to trace your number in the air.

• Make it tiny and huge.

• Draw it above, below and behind your body.

• Trace your number with your elbow, knee, toes, back, head or other body part. Make small and gigantic numbers.

Then encourage each child to try drawing several numbers using various body parts.

Entire Body

• Use your whole body to make your number.

• Imagine your entire body has paint on it.

• Move through the space while painting the curvy and straight lines of your number.

Then ask students to try tracing several numbers using their entire body.

Count to 10

Locomotor Steps

• Move through the biggest amounts of space that you can cover by the time the teacher says, "Ten."

• Do the following for 10 counts: skip, slide, jump, hop, and gallop. Go as far as you can during the 10 counts.

Entire Body

• You have 10 counts to get larger and larger.

• Then take one count to get as small as possible. Repeat this several times varying the speed. For example: "You have nine counts to get bigger and one count to become tiny."

Good-Bye Dance for the Arithmetic Lesson

Count the Boxes

The group sits in a circle. Talk about what we worked on today.

- Each child takes a turn picking up an imaginary box. Designate which child is performing. The group will keep track of the number of boxes by counting out loud.

Start the Good-Bye Dance

- Pick up a small, light box and carry it to a place in the room. Put it down.

- Lift huge, heavy boxes and build onto the other boxes.

- Jump, skip, slide and gallop your box around the room. Place it on the pile of other boxes.

- Push and then pull your heavy box.

- What was the total number of our boxes?

You may wish to use the boxes for teaching addition or subtraction.

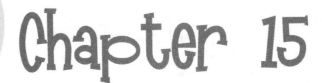

Elements of Movement:

Space: Pathways
Shape: Big/Little
Kinetics: Rhythm

Chapter 15

Trains

The group should sit in a circle. Discuss different modes of transportation. Talk about vehicles of transportation. Name vehicles with wheels or vehicles that travel in the water. Lead a conversation about the people who work in the transportation business. Help students share ideas about where people go. Use the following prompts:

• One time I flew in an airplane, rode in a train, bus, car . . .

• On my vacation I . . .

• In my suitcase I have . . .

Preparation

• Place many colored pieces of tape on the floor. Make an X with each piece of tape. Keep lots of space between the Xs.

Draw the following patterns on the chalkboard:

• Figure eight, square, triangle, diamond, spiral and serpentine shapes.

Start the Lesson

Body Parts on your "Self-Space"

• Shake and wiggle your fingers, hands, wrists, elbows, shoulders, head, nose, ribs, hips, knees, legs, ankles and feet.

• Shake your entire body.

Warm Up in Place

- Use your hands to pat your arms, hands, shoulders, neck, head, back, ribs, tummy, hips, legs, ankles and feet.

- Pat your whole body.

Locomotion

- Chug your train fast and slow throughout the room. *Repeat several times.*

- Accompany slow movements with "chug, chug, chug, chug . . ."

- Accompany fast, explosive movements into space with "whoo, whoo . . ."

- Become a wavy train using your arms and back.

- Rock your wavy train using high and low levels in space.

- Shuffle your train with changing levels—high, medium and low.

- Stretch and reach your train into all of the directions around the body. Stretch above, below, behind, sideways and in front of you.

- Travel through the space as a bouncy train, a leisurely train, a lickety-split train, a shaking train, a wiggling train, a jerky train and a powerful train. Use your muscles to show the strength of your train.

- Run while tracing figure eights, squares, triangles, diamonds, spirals and serpentine floor patterns. You may have to change directions, stop and turn.

Repeat each shape several times.

Big and Little Shapes

Entire Body

• Point out the tape on the floor. Go find a train station to collapse on. Show me a collapsing train.

Explore the following contrasting small and big movements:

• Shrink slowly to a small shape.

• Stretch into a gigantic shape.

• Move fast into a tiny shape.

• Grow slowly into a wide shape.

• Melt into a low shape.

• Burst into an open shape.

• Close your body inward to a crouching position.

• Twirl into a twisted shape.

• Move smoothly into a bent shape.

• Fling yourself into a stretch.

• Drop into a sitting shape.

• Spin into a flat shape.

Good-Bye Dance for the Trains Lesson

The group sits in a circle. What elements of movement did we explore today? Divide the class in half. Find a partner in your group. Sit together on an X.

Start the Good-Bye Dance

- Freeze in a starting shape.

- Show your favorite moving train. You can choose some of the ways we moved today—chug, wavy and shuffle.

- You and your partner don't have to move the same way, but stay together.

- Freeze in an ending shape.

Give the other group a turn to perform.

- Gradually tap each child. Ask them to join other "dancing trains." Everybody helps to make one train. The train travels and freezes in a shape several times.

- Everyone becomes a slow, broken down, dilapidated train. Accompany the train while repeating *dilapidated* to end the class.

Chapter 16

Game Day

The activities in this chapter are for fun. Use these lessons on days when the children have a lot of energy or if there is extra time at the end of class. They can be inserted into any other curricula. Children need plenty of opportunities to explore their physical limits.

Locomotor Tag

Tag each child as the leader, thereby assuring each child has a turn. Everyone follows the leader's movements. Give students ample time to explore a starting shape, move through the space and create an ending shape.

• Freeze in a shape.

• Move that shape through the space.

• Freeze in a shape.

Tag the next child.

Body Part Talk

• Have a conversation between your hip and your foot, your ear and your ankle, etc.

Stick Together Body Parts

• Stick your elbow onto your knee. Find a way to move through space. Continue calling out body parts to stick together and discover how to travel through space.

Stick Together with a Partner

Body Parts

- Stick your elbows, knees, back, hip, fingers and toes together.

Locomotor Movements

- Find ways to move while staying connected to your partner.

- Move in straight/curvy pathways, high/low levels and free flowing. Also try bound, controlled movements while stuck together. Explore each of the elements of movement.

Alphabet Group Dance

Locomotor Steps and Frozen Shapes

Pick a starting location at one end of the room. Bring students together in this area. Children perform one at a time. Tap a child. He or she will then travel to the other side of the room using a locomotor step such as a run, skip, gallop or slide. The student will freeze in a shape at the other end of the room. This will gradually become a group shape. Everyone will say the alphabet together as each child moves. Call out different locomotor steps for the Alphabet Dance.

- Everyone says "A" together. One child runs and then freezes in a shape.

- Everyone calls out "B." The next child skips and then freezes in a shape near the first child.

- Everyone says "C." The next child gallops and freezes with the other children, etc.

- Everyone takes a turn. Begin again until you finish the alphabet. On "Z" the class melts their "group shape" onto the floor.

Traffic Lights

• Place the following words on the chalkboard. The teacher calls out:

Red: "Stop,"

Green: "Skip forward"

Yellow: "Walk in place," etc.

Red	Green	Yellow
Stop	Skip Forward	Walk in Place
Sit	Gallop	Spin on Bottoms
Upside Down Shape	High Tiptoe	Crawl
Freeze in a Shape	Floppy Walk	Shake in Place
Twisted Shape	Giant Steps	Tiny Ball Shape
Run in Place	Straight-Legged Walk	Flat, Low Shape
Rock	Curvy Walk	Stare
Collapsing	Balance on One Leg	Wide Shape
Hopping in Place	Roll	Angular Shape
Spring Up in Place	Jumping	Folded-Up Shape
Turn in Place	Run in Curvy Paths	
	Slide	

Traffic Light Dance

- Each child picks his own movements for the red, green and yellow traffic signals. Call out, "red, green or yellow." *Repeat this activity several times.*

Non-Locomotor Movements Staying in Place

Divide the class into two groups. Each group makes a big circle. The hot energy ball is in the center of each circle. The entire class performs each of the following movements:

- Bend the hot energy ball, twist it, shake it, rock it, jump with it, hop with it, stamp on it, turn it, collapse with it, spin it and stretch it. Keep it moving: it's hot!

- Repeat with half the class as the audience. Give both groups a turn to perform.

Paint the Air with Body Parts

- Put imaginary paint on your elbow. Flick paint toward the corner of the room. Ready, go!

- Continue choosing body parts and parts of the room.

- End with paint on your entire body.

- Paint the entire room

- Finish by wiping, sweeping and flicking the paint off until you're clean.

Mirrors

Divide students into partners. One child leads the movement exploration while the other follows. The leader can move any way he or she wants. The other child faces his or her partner and imitates the movements like a mirror reflection. Change roles.

Lesson Reviews:

The Visual Aid Guide Boxes

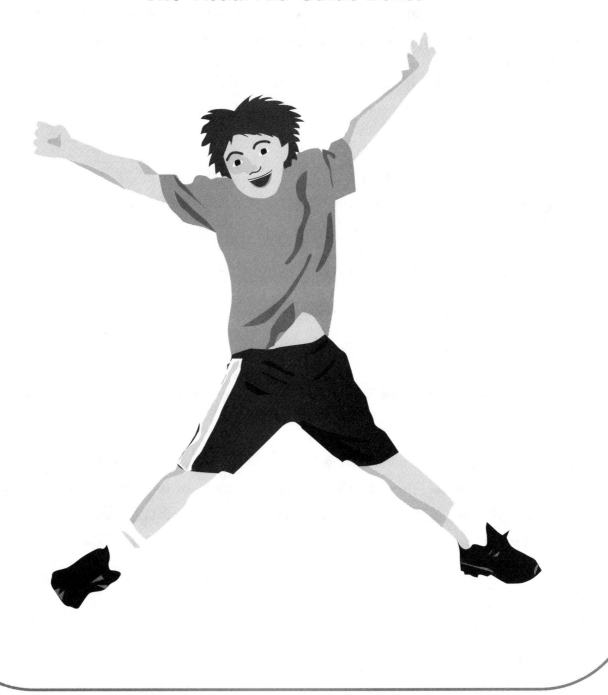

Chapter 2: Laying the Groundwork Lesson

Write the words below on the chalkboard. This is a summary of the lesson.

Once is not enough. Give the children plenty of time to explore each direction. Let them repeat the movements several times.

Name Rhythms

Clap each child's name several times.

Room and Spatial Orientation

- Stretch your elbows while moving to the window.

- Shake your stomachs while traveling to the door.

- Lead with your back while moving to the chalkboard.

Repeat several times, changing body parts and room destinations.

Explore Your Own "Self-Space"

1. Locomotor Moves

• Find your own X on the floor. This is your "Self-Space." Stretch as far as you can in every direction without leaving your X.

• Jump on your spot.

• Run in place as fast as you can on your spot.

• Run slowly on the X.

• Find as many ways as you can to leap over your spot.

• Turn and twist on your X.

• Try turns and spins on high, medium and low levels.

• Hop on your spot changing legs, then in different ways.

2. Body Parts

• Put your hand, bottom, back, belly, toes, elbows, top of your head and other parts of your body on your "Self-Space" while stretching the rest of your body away.

• Put your foot, etc., on your X and then move it as far away as you can. Try this again with your ear, arm, belly, hand, etc.

• Lead with your elbow, knee, head, etc., all over your "Self-Space." Don't move away from it.

• Move a body part around, over and across your X.

• Circle a body part above, behind and below while moving high and low.

• Find exciting ways to surround your X.

Movement and stillness

- Move quickly and suddenly freeze.

- Shake your body as fast as you can and then freeze.

- Hold your shape while I take a picture with an imaginary camera.

- Try another shape, and another . . .

- Move slowly and freeze like a statue.

Repeat this several times changing the look of your statue.

- Try curled, wide and gnarled statue shapes, adding frozen moments.

Chapter 3: Explore the Basics Lesson

Take an imaginary piece of chalk out of the air.

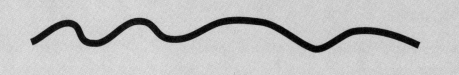

straight and Curvy Lines on your spot

- Trace straight lines above, below, behind and in front of you. Try small and large movements.

- Trace curvy lines above, below, behind and in front of you.

- Trace curvy lines above you and suddenly freeze in a round shape. Begin to trace curvy lines again. Freeze in another circular shape.

- Trace circles and form the shape of a circle with your body. Periodically "freeze" in that shape before continuing to trace circles again.

Zip, Chucka, Dot Dance

- Take an imaginary piece of chalk out of the air.

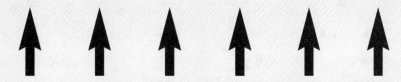

- Say "Zip" repetitively, while moving from a low to a high level. Trace the chalk lines from low to high several times. Also try starting from a crouched position. Explode upwards into jumps.

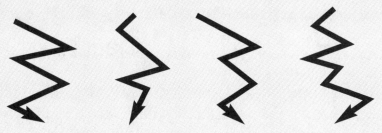

- While gradually moving the body downward repeat, "Chucka, chucka, chucka" and draw sharp chalk lines. Rise again. Repeat this activity several times.

- Designate different points in space while saying, "Dot, dot, dot . . ."
- Move the body on high, medium and low levels.
- Try placing the dots in front of you, to your right, to your left, behind, above and below you.
- Combine the "zip," "chucka" and "dot" movements.

Curvy, Zigzag and Straight Pathways

- Skip, run, walk, gallop and slide, while adding frozen round or straight shapes.

- Run, walk, gallop, jump and slide in curvy and straight pathways.

- Draw huge zigzag lines in front of you.

- Use your feet to trace small and big zigzag lines on the floor.

- Walk, run, skip and slide in small and big curvy lines on the floor.

The "EE" "OO" "AA" Dance

- Find an X on the floor.

- Make narrow, wide and bent shapes on a high level while making the sound, "EE."

- Try different wide shapes on a medium level that stretch forward, backwards, sideways and balance on one leg—while making the sound "OO."

- Perform round and flat shapes on a low level in the space while making the sound "AA."

- Combine these moves several times. Try a high stretch on "EE," a wide stretch on "OO" and a low bend on "AA."

Chapter 4: Locomotor Movements

The group begins by sitting in a circle.

Locomotor steps: 1

- Look up, down, right, left, behind you, at your neighbor, into the circle and away from the circle. Imagine you can put "eyes" on your nose. Get up and run around the room, leading with your nose.

- Skip high while leading with your knees.

- Jump, leading with the top of your head.

- Slide, leading from your hips while changing directions.

- Run through the space leading with your chest. Run in place. Run backwards leading with your bottom.

- Turn while leading with your elbows.

- Try walking very low while making sharp changes of direction. Lead with your feet.

Locomotor steps: 2

- Begin at one end of the room. Move to the other side of the room.

- Run, walk, skip, jump, gallop, hop, slide, leap, giant steps, tiptoe and roll to the other side of the room.

- Move throughout the space while exploring these steps: high walk, silly walk, stiff march, bouncy walk, floating, stargazing, heavy walk, jerky walk, slow-motion walk, stroll, shaky walk, hobble, backwards walk, sideways walk, curvy walk and straight walk.

Invent New steps

Try a cross-legged walk, duck walk, heel-slapping walk, straight- legged walk, knee lifts, bear walk, jumping jacks, inch-worms, rabbit jumps and crab walk.

Chapter 5: Bones Lesson

Body Parts
- Move and circle your bones.

Entire Body
- Twist, bend, stretch and turn.

Locomotor Movements
- Imagine you can move using only your bones and joints in the following ways: tiptoe, floppy, wiggle, shake, hobble, drag, melt, spin, roll, rise, prance, march, kick, leap, whip and fling.

- Move fast/slow and high/low with rattling and creaky bones.

- Jog, skip, jump, gallop and slide.

Chapter 6: Buildings, Subways and Drawbridges Lesson
Explore Big and Little Locomotor Steps

Running
- Tiny runs on your "Self-Space."
- Run without traveling very much.
- Run covering a lot of space.

Skipping
- Tiny skips and wide skips.

Galloping
- Gallop on your "Self-Space."
- Make your gallops bigger and bigger.
- Freeze in a wide, stretched-out shape.

Jumping
- Small jumps in place.
- Tiny jumps that travel.
- Big, wide, springy jumps into the space.

Tiptoe steps
- Tiny and wide tiptoe steps.

Slides

- Tiny and big slides.

Subways and Tunnels

- Use body parts and the entire body to make small and large tunnels.

- Tiny tunnels grow bigger and vice versa.

Round and Pointed Buildings

- Use your entire body to make buildings.

- Make tall, thin, wide, round and pointed buildings.

- Move the buildings through space.

Drawbridges

- Make bridge shapes with your body.

- Open the drawbridge by lifting different body parts.

Chapter 7: Beanbags and Rocks Lesson

Shaking

- Sitting and standing, shake your fingers, hands, toes, feet, belly, back and entire body like a beanbag.

- Designate different body parts to shake up high, down low, in front and at either side of the body.

- Stand and shake the entire body on a high level. Shake your body on a low level.

- Try small shakes while lying down using your toes, ankles, legs, hands and arms.

- Sit and shake your arms in big, slow movements forward, backwards and sideways.

- Travel in the room and turn whenever you want while shaking.

- Jump and twirl with imaginary beanbags inside you.

Investigate the smooth shapes of Rocks

- Can you turn your body into the shape of a round rock?

- Try small and large rock-like shapes.

- Use your upper body to make circles above, below and behind you.

Take your rock shapes for a run.

- Change directions forward and backwards.

- Trace circular pathways along the floor.

- How many ways can you skip, run, slide, swing, rise and collapse in circles?

Heavy and Light Movements

- Imagine picking up rocks and putting them in a bucket.

- Grab light, tiny rocks while walking, tiptoeing, turning and running fast.

- Gather gigantic rocks while dragging, leaning, pushing and pulling them.

- Drag your heavy bucket.

- Dump the rocks out of the bucket using all of your muscles.

- Shake any extra rocks out of the bucket.

Beanbag Dance

- Give each child a beanbag.

- Balance the beanbag on your hand, shoulder, head, knee, etc.

- Travel while balancing the beanbag on various body parts.

- Move high, low, crouch, turn and tiptoe while balancing the beanbag on different body parts.

- Rise, travel and collapse whenever the beanbag falls.

Repeat this activity several times. Find different ways to rise, balance, travel and collapse with the beanbag.

Chapter 8: Meteorites Lesson

Breathing
- Use your entire body.

- Make big and small shapes while sitting and standing. Slowly rise, stretch and collapse.

Sigh
- Entire body: short, smooth, rise and fall.

- Body parts: sigh with your elbow, ear and foot.

- Locomotion: take your sigh for a walk, skip, run and jump.

Hiccup
- Tiny, quick, jerky, rise and fall.

- Entire body: springy jumps low/medium/high level and light turns.

- Body parts: hiccup your shoulder, eye, neck, finger and back.

Sneeze

- Entire body with rhythms: sustained with percussive, strong, fast collapse.

- Rhythms: short, fast, strong and percussive.

- Body parts: feel the sneeze in your spine, etc.

- Locomotion: huge sneeze while running from one end of the room to the other.

- Traveling backwards say "Ahhhhh," running forward say "Chooo."

Meteorites

- Shake it high, low and with frozen moments.

- Circle, high/low, slow/fast, above and behind.

- Combine high and low levels with long, sustained and short, percussive movements.

- Locomotion: Float, collapsing your upper body.

- Rise, jump, run, turn and collapse in a low shape.

- Throw it up near you and imitate it.

- Soar through space, move like it did, rising and collapsing.

Empty Suit of Clothes Dance

Body Parts

Curl your body into the smallest shape possible and then stretch like a rubber band. Use the following body parts:

- Fingers, hands, wrists, arms, elbows, bottoms, legs, knees, ankles, heels and toes.

- Arm/leg, neck/back, finger/toe and leg/head.

Entire Body

- Shrink into a narrow shape, stretch into a wide shape. Curl into a small shape and then grow into a flat, low, wide and high shape.

Moving Across the Room

- Stretch like an imaginary rubber band . . . run. Stretch it and gallop, stretch it and jump, stretch it and skip, stretch it and twirl, stretch it and floppy walk and stretch it and take giant steps.

- Imagine shooting a rubber band. Now do that with your whole body.

Butterfly Dance

Chapter 10: Pathways Lesson

Take an imaginary piece of paper and a crayon from the air.

Body Parts

- Draw curvy lines with different body parts.

- Draw straight lines using your nose, elbow, back or other body part.

Entire Body

- Make curvy round shapes using your whole body.
- Trace curvy lines by swinging, circling, turning, twisting, spinning and rolling.
- Trace straight lines.
- Make straight, angular shapes several times while freezing the shapes.

Locomotor Movements

- Everyone help roll a huge piece of imaginary paper out along the floor space.

- Find **straight** shapes with your body.

- Put imaginary paint on your feet. Trace straight lines all over the imaginary paper on the floor. Dash and dart through the space. Take sharp corners and make abrupt stops.

- Move while making razor-like, angular shapes with your body.

- Run, walk or skip in straight pathways.

- Make sharp changes of directions forward, backward, sideways and turning around corners.

- Freeze in an angular shape.

Jump when the teacher removes the piece of paper. Everyone spreads a new imaginary sheet of paper across the floor.

- Find **curvy** shapes.

- Trace tiny and big curvy lines throughout the space.

- Run in curvy pathways while leaning your body to the left and to the right.

- Change directions by moving backwards, sideways and turning.

- Add curvy shapes to your body while changing directions.

Jump when the paper is removed. Then roll out a new sheet of imaginary paper.

- Make **curvy** and **straight** shapes with your body.

- Locomote through space tracing curvy and straight pathways.

- Move forward, backwards and sideways in straight and curvy paths.

Jump when the paper is removed. Now trace curvy and straight pathways while:

- Squishing into sand, dashing across hot sand, splashing through water, sinking into mud and skittering along the sidewalk without stepping on the cracks.

Trace curvy and straight pathways wearing hiking boots.

- Move in jerky movements, powerful, heavy, staggering, dragging, chugging, pounding and climbing.

Trace curvy and straight pathways wearing moccasins.

- Move quietly, softly, smoothly, crouching, brushing, fast and gently.

Make curvy and straight pathways wearing cowboy boots.

- Perform kicks, gallops, jumps, turns, leaps and struts.

Trace curvy and straight pathways wearing flippers.

- Move as if you were flicking, sinking, waving, whipping, flinging and cross-legged steps.

Make curvy and straight pathways while wearing pointed elf shoes.

- Move brightly, sharply, dart, tap, wiggle and perform tiny jumps.

Chapter 11: Statues Lesson

Frozen Shapes

- Begin sitting in a group on the floor. Notice that your body is making a particular sitting shape. It is different from the person next to you. On the count of 3, sit in a different shape. Repeat several times. Also try lying down and standing shapes.

- Skip across the room and freeze in a curled shape.

- Jump around the room and freeze in a high, narrow shape.

- Gallop and end in a wide, stretched-out shape.

- Slide and end in a twisted shape.

- Run and end in a low, flat shape.

- Roll and finish in a round ball.

- Walk backwards and end in an upside-down shape.

Freeze and Move

- Make a tiny shape. Freeze it. Move it all over the space. Try other round, curled and narrow shapes.

- Find gigantic, puffed up, circular, towering, crouched and wide shapes.

- Freeze in each shape and then move them around the room.

Flying Shapes

- Divide the class in half. Jump into the air. Move over the line of tape you placed across the center of the room.

- Freeze in a starting shape.

- Run and jump over the line of tape.

- Make a stretched-out shape while you are in the air.

- End on the other side of the room in a frozen shape.

Perform the following airborne shapes:
- Turning, tiny, gigantic, narrow, curvy, bent, low, wide-legged, twisted, backwards and collapsed.

You may also want them to explore flying into the air like a skier going over a jump, a hot air balloon, an ice skater, a kite, an airplane, a bird, a cloud and an astronaut.

Clay

- Make tiny, round, wide, curvy, straight, twisted and flat clay shapes.

- Move like heavy clay.

- Jump, run, slide or gallop like heavy clay.

Wire

- Perform twisted, stretched, sharp, straight, corkscrew and spiraling wire shapes.

- Take your wire shapes for a run.

- Spring into wire shapes.

- Feel your wire shapes changing into clay and vice versa.

Statues and Sculptors

Chapter 12: Pick a Word Lesson

- Make two sets of cards before class.

- Place the locomotor movement words on one set of cards. Make several cards containing the following locomotor steps: **skip, walk, run, gallop, jump, slide** and **hop.**

- Place the action words on another set of cards. Make several cards containing the following action words: **push, big, heavy, zigzag, high, off-balance, prickly, join, soar, halt, sticky, pause, grinning** and **mingle.**

- Each child chooses a locomotor step card.

Movements

- Explore your locomotor step: **skip, walk, run, gallop, jump, slide or hop**.

Add the following variations to the locomotor step you chose:

- **Level changes:** high/medium/low.

- **Directions:** forward/backwards/sideways.

- **Size:** small/large.

- **Speed:** fast/slow.

- **Force:** light/heavy.

For example: show your step high and then low. Change directions forward, backwards and sideways. Explore tiny steps. Take up a lot of space with gigantic steps. Move fast and in slow motion. Step as light as a feather and then make heavy steps.

Action Words

- Each child chooses an action word card. Explore your action word in any way you choose.

- Combine the action words with running.

- Give them plenty of opportunities to explore the following action words: **push, big, heavy, zigzag, high, off-balance, prickly, join, soar, halt, sticky, pause, grinning and mingle while running**.

- Run while pushing something.

- Run taking up large amounts of space.

- Show me a heavy run.

- Run in zigzag pathways.

- Try high runs that fall off-balance.

- Explore running with a prickly sensation along your spine.

- Join a classmate while running.

- Find ways to make airborne shapes. Soar through the air like a kite.

- Run and abruptly stop.

- Run through sticky taffy and pause several times.

- Mingle with your classmates while grinning.

If time permits, repeat the directions above with other locomotor steps.

Chapter 13: Places and Environments Lesson

Body Parts
- Curl your toes, fingers, arms or back.

- Stretch each body part.

Rain Puddles
- Take huge, wide steps.

- Balance on one leg while moving over the puddles.

- Jump into the water or hop on the puddles.

- Shuffle through the water or dash across the puddles.

Mud
1. Body Parts
Keep naming a body part that is stuck in the mud.

- Stretch . . . stretch . . . stretch away using the rest of your body.

2. Locomotion
- Move heavily through the mud.

- Step high out of the mud while shaking the dirt off of your feet.

- Tiny gallops and stretched-out gallops through the mud.

Marshmallows

- Smoothly, lightly, spring up, tiptoe, twirl, bounce, float, ooze, collapse, roll and somersault.

- Melt and rise several times.

On Ice

- Balance, fall, fast, slow, smooth, slide, soar, push, glide and spin on your bottom or belly.

- Sway and slide side-to-side, forward and backwards.

Hot sand

- Dance with accents that are jerky, sharp, jagged and angular.

- Squish your toes into the sand.

- Spring, jump, hop and kick high.

Buzzing Bees

- Run fast while swinging and swatting.

- Dart, swing, shake, swat, wiggle, flick, scratch, stomp, duck, swirl and lean.

- Move low and fast with your mouth tightly closed.

Sleeping Cats

- Creep, crawl, tiptoe, slide and sway.

- Pat and rub the cats.

- Stop quietly while curling and uncurling.

- Take wide, soft steps around and over the cats.

Pit Full of Snakes

- Move cautiously around the snakes on low, medium and high levels.

- Bravely run, dodge, jump and leap over the snakes.

- Make twisted, tiny and flat shapes traveling in curvy paths.

- Travel backwards while looking over your shoulder.

Chapter 14: Arithmetic Lesson

Body Parts

- Find a number on the floor.

- Place your hands, elbow, ear, etc., on the number. Stretch the rest of your body away from the number.

- Trace your number in the air using your finger. Make it tiny and huge. Draw it above, below and behind your body.

- Draw your number with your elbow, knee, toes, back, head or other body part. Make it small and gigantic.

- Encourage them to try drawing several numbers using body parts.

Entire Body

- Put imaginary paint on your entire body.

- Move all over the space while painting the curvy and straight lines of your number.

Try several numbers.

Count to 10

1. Steps

- Move through the biggest amounts of space that you can cover by the time the teacher counts to 10.

- You have 10 counts to skip, slide, jump, hop and gallop. Travel as far as you can during the 10 counts.

2. Entire Body

- Take 10 counts to get larger and larger.
- In one count, make your body as small as possible. Repeat this several times. Now you have nine counts to get bigger and one count to become tiny.

Chapter 15: Trains Lesson

Body Parts

- Shake and wiggle your fingers, hands, wrists, elbows, shoulders, head, nose, ribs, hips, knees, legs, ankles and feet.

- Shake your entire body.

Warm Up

- Use your hands to pat your arms, hands, shoulders, neck, head, back, ribs, tummy, hips, legs, ankles and feet.

- Pat your whole body.

Locomotion

- Chug your train fast and slow throughout the entire room.

- Move slowly saying, "Chug, chug, chug, chug . . ."

- Explode fast into the space saying, "Whoo, whoo . . ."

- Wavy train. Rock your wavy train while changing levels—high, medium and low.

- Shuffle your train, changing levels.

- Stretch and reach your train into all of the directions around your body. Stretch above, below, behind, sideways and in front of you.

- Bouncing train, leisurely train, lickety-split train, shaking train, wiggling train, jerky train and a powerful train.

Trace

- Figure eights, squares, triangles, diamonds, spirals and serpentine floor patterns. Repeat each one several times.

- Run with changes of direction, stops and turns.

Big and Little shapes

- Point out the tape on the floor.

- Become a collapsing train. Find a train station to collapse on. Children collapse on the pieces of tape.

Perform the following contrasting big and small movements:
- Shrink slowly into a small shape.

- Stretch into a gigantic shape.

- Move fast into a tiny shape.

- Grow slowly into a wide shape.

- Melt into a low shape.

- Burst into an open shape.

- Close your body inward into a crouched position.

- Twirl into a twisted shape.

- Move smoothly into a bent shape.

- Fling yourself into a stretch.

- Drop into a sitting shape.

- Spin into a flat shape.

127

Create healthy habits for adults with the ABC exercises in Functional Fitness

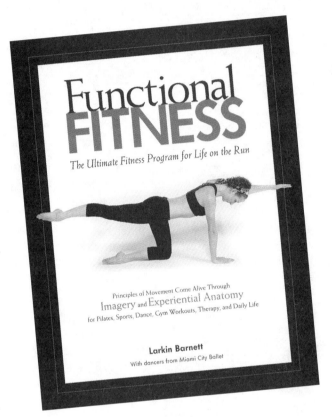

Functional Fitness:
The Ultimate Fitness Program
for Life on the Run

By Larkin Barnett

With dancers from Miami City Ballet

Available at:
www.Amazon.com
www.FloridaAcademicPress.com
www.FitSimply.com

Design and illustrations by Kristen Bergman Morales

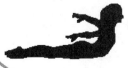

Copyright © 2008 Larkinetics®

www.FitSimply.com